RISK AND RECOVERY: AIDS, HIV AND ALCOHOL

About the Authors

Marcia Quackenbush, MS, MFCC (Marriage, Family, and Child Counselor) has worked at the AIDS Health Project since its founding in 1984. She has counseled individuals and facilitated groups for people coping with HIV disease, and has trained teachers, and mental health and other health providers throughout the country about HIV-related issues. She is the co-editor of *The AIDS Challenge: Prevention Education for Young People* (ETR Associates: 1988) and co-author of *"Does AIDS Hurt?" Educating Young Children About AIDS* (ETR Associates, second edition 1992).

JD Benson, MS, MFCC is Senior Trainer for the Provider Training Program at the AIDS Health Project. She has been involved in agency-based, as well as private, HIV-related counseling, training, and consultation since 1985, and has co-authored several training curricula about HIV disease for mental health counselors, antibody test counselors and their trainers, and alcohol recovery home staff. Her work with the alcohol recovery community has included recovery groups for women as well as individual, couples, and family counseling. Ms. Benson is a founder of the East Bay Women's AIDS Network (WAN) and a board member of San Francisco WAN.

Joanna Rinaldi Is Program Director of the AIDS Health Project Hospital Services Unit at San Francisco General Hospital. She has worked in the substance abuse field for more than 10 years and has focused on HIV disease since 1986, delivering aggressive intervention services to substance users with HIV disease and producing HIV-related professional training for providers. She was the coordinator of the project's AIDS and Substance Abuse Program and the co-author of *AIDS and Substance Abuse: A Training Manual for Health Care Professionals.*

Gary James Wood, JD, who wrote the majority of Chapter 7: *Legal Issues for Providers,* is Principal Attorney at AIDS Legal Consultants. He co-founded the world's largest AIDS Legal Referral Panel in San Francisco, lectures and publishes widely, and provides HIV-related technical assistance to organizations. He is a co-author of *AIDS Law for Mental Health Professionals (Updated Version)*, published 1992 by the AIDS Health Project.

RISK AND RECOVERY

AIDS, HIV AND ALCOHOL

A Handbook for Providers

Marcia Quackenbush, MFCC
JD Benson, MFCC
with Joanna Rinaldi

Published by
The AIDS Health Project
University of California San Francisco

Distributed to the Trade by
Celestial Arts
Berkeley, California

For Information and comments: UCSF AIDS Health Project, Box 0884, San Francisco, California 94143-0884.

For Trade Discounts and Returns: Celestial Arts, P. O. Box 7327, Berkeley California, 94707.

The AIDS Health Project is an affiliated unit of the Langley Porter Psychiatric Institute, School of Medicine, University of California San Francisco.

First Printing, October 1992. Printed in the United States of America

Library of Congress Cataloging-in-Publication Data
Quackenbush, Marcia.
Risk and Recovery : AIDS, HIV and Alcohol : a handbook for providers / Marcia Quackenbush, JD Benson with Joanna Rinaldi.
p. cm.
Includes bibliographical references and index.
ISBN 0–89087–690–8 : $16.95
1. HIV infections—Prevention. 2. Alcoholics—Rehabilitation. 3. Alcoholism counseling. I. Benson, JD, 1953– . II. Rinaldi, Joanna. III. Title.
RO644.A25Q3 1992 92-26635
616.97'9205—dc20 CIP

UCSF AIDS Health Project Publications

James W. Dilley, MD	Director, AIDS Health Project
Robert Marks	Publications Manager, Editor
Paul Causey, Richard McCormack	Marketing and Outreach
Saul Rosenfield	Design, Computer Templates
Sayre Van Young	Indexing
Leslie Samuels	Production
Kathy Barr, E. Miguel Thurman, Roger Scroggs	Proofreading
Sandra Kriletich	Distribution
Saul Rosenfield, JD Benson	Cover Design
Marcia Quackenbush	Text Illustrations

John Tighe, Dorothy Stinnett, Clare Potter, Suzanne Papakonstantinou, Hazel Garcia provided editorial and production assistance. JoAnn Uchida and Roger Scroggs provided fiscal and administrative support.

Donations: The computer fonts used in this book were donated by *Adobe Systems,* Mountain View, California. The linotronic plates for its production were partially donated by *Design & Type,* San Francisco. We thank these companies for their generosity.

CONTENTS

PREFACE

Since 1984, the AIDS Health Project, a program of the University of California San Francisco, has developed mental health programs for people with HIV disease and those at risk for infection. The project serves more than 20,000 clients a year, and has trained more than 20,000 providers throughout California. The project also offers a broad range of other services, including an AIDS and Substance Abuse Program, which directly addresses HIV-related issues for active and recovering alcoholics and drug addicts.

Because of our experience in this area, we were invited in 1989 to write a training on HIV disease and alcohol for providers working in licensed alcohol recovery homes in California. The Office of Alcohol and Drug Problems (OADP) of the California Department of Health Services extended this offer and funded the project.

An Advisory Group of providers and experts from throughout California was assembled, and with the help of their feedback, we designed two trainings, one for administrators in the recovery home system, the other for front-line providers. These trainings were field-tested and then offered in 1990 and 1991 to representatives of 68 recovery agencies throughout the state.

This experience proved to us that there was an interest and a need for accurate, relevant, and clear information about HIV disease and alcohol. One of the strengths of the training project was its presentation of HIV-related information in a context consistent with the theoretical framework of alcohol recovery providers themselves, especially the principles and practice of Alcoholics Anonymous.

ACKNOWLEDGMENTS

Many people contributed ideas and information for this book. The willingness of providers and participants in recovery to share their experiences and impressions has resulted in a richer and more comprehensive work. We thank everyone who helped during the design, testing, and provision of the original HIV and Alcohol Training Project, as well as those who have offered suggestions about the text of this book.

In particular, we would like to thank Mary Huttner, formerly of the California OADP, for following through on an early vision and contacting us about the original training. We would also like to thank the members of the Advisory Group for that project: Peggy Barnett, Jerry DeJong, Laurie Drabble, Douglas Gibbs, Diane Grey, Joanne Lovejoy, Bernadine Luckey, Russ Mills, Sharon Ng, Carol Nottley, Virginia Saldana-Grove, Helen Waukazoo, and Jeff Wynne. Michael Caron of OADP provided thoughtful monitoring.

Several individuals took time to read early drafts of this book and offered us excellent suggestions for improvement. Thank you Robert Paul Cabaj, MD, Jeanie Dobbs, Jerry DeJong, and Carol Nottley. Ellen Dayton reviewed concepts and materials during each stage of the writing. James W. Dilley, MD, Executive Director of the AIDS Health Project, made it possible for staff to put time and effort into this project and provided thoughtful review of the text.

Gary James Wood, JD, graciously shared his legal expertise with us in Chapter 7: *Legal Issues for Providers.* We are lucky to benefit from his knowledge. Noel Day, President of Polaris Research and Development, contributed substantially to the concepts about cultural norms and differences in Chapter 6: *Culture and Attitude.*

Thank you to Rob Marks, our meticulous editor, and Saul Rosenfield, who gave much time to the design of the book.

Finally, we offer a special thank you to participants and providers in recovery who have made a commitment to address the issue of HIV disease and alcohol. In so doing, they are taking steps to save lives, to support sobriety, and to welcome and give comfort to people with HIV disease in recovery.

Personal Acknowledgments

Thank you to family, friends, and colleagues who have supported my work on this project; to those special friends who, through their experience, strength, and hope, have helped me learn about the family disease of alcoholism; and to Mark R., who showed me some of the ways a strong program of recovery could help an alcoholic with HIV disease.

– Marcia Quackenbush

How we arrive at our conclusions, and the quality of that process, is often of greater significance to me than the conclusions we may reach. In this instance, the conclusion is a book that I hope will be of assistance to some, if not all, who read it.

I wish to acknowledge Aelsa Steckel, a therapist, and Rhonda C., both of SF Bay area. Each in her own way, and long ago, shared her compassion and courage at a turning point in my healing journey.

I thank Marcia Quackenbush and JoAnna Rinaldi, sometimes for their ardor, sometimes for their silence, as ideas were formulated and reworked, and as the wordsmithing progressed. As three women authoring one book together, I am hopeful that our diversity of life experience will complement our common lives as women, enriching the text.

As Saul Rosenfield and I explored cover design ideas, the boundary between work and play dissolved. I thank him.

I wish to thank my life partner, Mindy S. Benson, PNP. She took time to listen to my ideas and to review matters relevant to perinatal transmission and pediatric HIV disease. Finally, I want to thank our son Seth for being the light of my life, and my Higher Power for revealing the beauty and kindness there is in living.

– JD Benson

IMPORTANT TERMS

Although we have included a glossary in this book, there are several terms used throughout the text that are important either because they are essential to understanding the material or because they have special definitions in the context of this book.

Recovery

"Recovery" is a process by which alcoholics or people with addictions can actively address and change attitudes and behaviors. It is a lifelong process; alcoholics can be "in recovery" but are never "recovered." Individuals seeking recovery through the 12-step model of Alcoholics Anonymous develop a way of living which, when applied one day at a time, can diminish or eliminate the compulsion to engage in drinking or other behaviors.

This may be accomplished by attending 12-step meetings, reading 12-step literature, and learning from the "experience, strength, and hope" of others in recovery. In addition, service is an important part of recovery, and may include sharing with others what it was like before recovery, what precipitated the beginning of the recovery process, and how recovery has gone, as well as more practical approaches like helping with meeting tasks.

Provider

"Provider" includes private practitioners in mental health or counseling and individuals working in formal recovery settings (recovery homes, inpatient hospital units, and outpatient programs), in mental health settings (inpatient, outpatient, and day treatment programs), and in community-based outreach or service organizations.

Participant

Alcoholics addressing their disease through the Twelve Steps are active participants in the recovery process. In this book, "participant" designates people in recovery receiving some sort of supportive services. This may include residents in inpatient recovery programs, people in outpatient recovery programs, clients of agencies or programs that do not focus specifically on recovery issues, or individuals being seen in private counseling or psychotherapy.

Program

"Program" designates settings other than private practice, in which a participant might receive services. This includes alcohol recovery agencies or programs, mental health agencies, community based organizations, and hospital programs. In some instances, the term refers to a program of recovery, based on the Twelve Steps of Alcoholics Anonymous.

HIV disease, HIV infection, AIDS

The human immunodeficiency virus ("HIV") is the virus that causes AIDS. Anyone who has been infected with HIV is said to have "HIV disease" or "HIV infection." People with HIV infection may look and feel fine or may be quite sick. "HIV disease" refers to the full spectrum of HIV infection including: people who have no symptoms; people who have mild to moderate symptoms, but who do not meet the criteria for "AIDS" as defined by the federal government; and people with "AIDS," who do meet these criteria. AIDS is diagnosed when a person with HIV infection develops one or more specific HIV-related illnesses.

INTRODUCTION

The recovery field has experienced remarkable growth over the past 10 years. Providers working in recovery, mental health, and other settings have seen an ever-widening population of people seeking support through the use of the 12-step model of Alcoholics Anonymous (AA) and other programs. A knowledge of the principles and practice of 12-step programs has become an important clinical tool for these providers.

Coincidentally, over the years that 12-step programs and philosophies have become widely used, the AIDS epidemic has burgeoned. AIDS has changed from a rare disease affecting a few thousand people to an epidemic of more than 10 million people worldwide. In the United States, the cumulative number of AIDS cases has grown from around 200 in 1981 to well over 200,000 in 1992; an estimated 1.5 million to 2 million people in the U.S. are currently HIV infected.

Alcohol and the Risk of HIV Infection

One of the primary ways HIV is transmitted is through the sharing of needles or other equipment during injection drug use. Most providers working with current and former injection drug users have, by now, gathered considerable experience with HIV disease. Providers working with people in alcohol recovery, however, have not generally considered HIV disease to be relevant to their work. Since alcohol use involves no exchange of blood or other risky body fluids, alcoholics in recovery do not seem, at first glance, to be at any particular risk for HIV infection.

On closer examination, though, it is clear that alcohol use is associated with higher levels of HIV-related risk behaviors, in particular, unsafe sex. Many recovering alcoholics have engaged in

HIV-related risk behaviors in the past—including unprotected sex with multiple partners, unprotected male-to-male sex, and needle sharing during injection drug use. Some are engaging in behaviors that continue to put them at risk; others will face choices about future behaviors that could be risky. Additionally, there will be individuals who do not succeed in a given recovery effort. When they relapse into active alcoholism, they may also participate in HIV-related risk behaviors often associated with drinking.

This book brings together information and suggestions that can assist alcohol recovery providers in addressing the HIV epidemic in their work settings. The material includes facts about HIV disease and the history of the epidemic, reviews HIV-related issues for people in alcohol recovery, and outlines strategies for implementing HIV-related policies and practices in recovery settings. The most important message the book seeks to communicate is: Attention to HIV-related concerns can save sobriety and lives.

12-Step Perspective

This book emphasizes a 12-step perspective and uses examples often based on the application of 12-step principles. We chose this particular approach for several reasons:

- It is our goal to present information related to HIV disease and alcohol use in a style that is consistent with the recovery and care philosophies held by many providers in the alcohol recovery field.
- HIV-related counseling and education with recovery participants is most successful if presented within a framework that is familiar and trustworthy. The 12-step approach is widely used and provides this comfortable framework.
- There is no other resource available addressing HIV-related issues for providers using the 12-step perspective.

This book does not aim to convert readers to a 12-step philosophy. It seeks, instead, to act as a resource for providers already using 12-step principles or interested in learning more about this approach. (See also Appendix A: *Overview of Alcoholics Anonymous.*)

In addition, the emphasis of this book is specifically on people whose primary addiction is alcoholism. With some adaptation, however, much of this material will be applicable to participants with other recovery focuses, for example, those who are using the Twelve Steps to address compulsive spending, overeating, or codependency. This material will be especially useful in work with recovering drug addicts who employ a 12-step approach to cope with their addiction. Much will also benefit members of drug treatment programs or communities that do not use the Twelve Steps.

Alcohol recovery providers must prepare themselves to address HIV-related issues with clients and program participants. Providers can offer essential HIV prevention information, help participants assess the risks and benefits of HIV antibody testing, and establish a compassionate and supportive environment for the HIV-infected individuals with whom they work. The importance of this effort cannot be overemphasized. HIV disease is in the recovery community today, and the time has come for alcohol recovery providers to take part in the effort to respond to the epidemic.

CHAPTER ONE

HIV AND ALCOHOL: WHAT'S THE CONNECTION?

IN THIS CHAPTER:

- HIV DISEASE: AN OVERVIEW
- ARE THERE PEOPLE WITH HIV DISEASE IN RECOVERY?
- HOW DO ALCOHOLICS GET HIV DISEASE?
- WHAT ARE THE FUTURE RISKS FOR PEOPLE IN RECOVERY?
- WHAT ISSUES ARISE WHEN PROVIDERS OR PARTICIPANTS HAVE HIV DISEASE?
- WHAT SHOULD RECOVERY PROVIDERS DO?
- WHAT ABOUT THE ALCOHOLIC WHO IS STILL USING?
- WHAT ABOUT THE "SOCIAL" DRINKER?
- WHAT'S THE CONNECTION?

CHAPTER ONE

HIV AND ALCOHOL: WHAT'S THE CONNECTION?

HIV Disease: An Overview

When AIDS was first described in 1981, little was known about the disease. Scientists were not sure what caused it, what behaviors put one at risk for it, or what steps could prevent it.

Today, knowledge about AIDS has come a long way. It is caused by a virus called HIV, or human immunodeficiency virus. HIV lives in blood, semen, and vaginal secretions. It is passed from person to person through sexual contact when partners share blood, semen or vaginal secretions or through some other exchange of blood or blood products. The best way to prevent the spread of HIV is to follow safer sex guidelines, so that blood, semen or vaginal secretions are not shared; and to avoid sharing needles or other equipment during injection drug use.*

AIDS prevention and education efforts have focused mainly on three groups:

- Injection drug users, some of whom have become infected with HIV by sharing needles or other paraphernalia (works).
- Sexual partners of injection drug users, some of whom have

* HIV can also live in other internal body fluids, such as those surrounding joints or organs, and in other body tissues. These substances are of concern to medical providers and emergency first aid workers. HIV can also be transmitted through organ transplants, which is why organ donors are usually screened for HIV infection. Outside of these specific medical situations, HIV transmission risks are generally limited to circumstances involving an exchange of blood, semen, or vaginal secretions.

become infected with HIV through unsafe sexual contact.

- Gay-identified men in urban areas, some of whom have become infected with HIV through unsafe sexual contact.

But information about HIV disease has not reached many people who need it, because education campaigns have either overlooked other populations or have presented information in ways that many people do not find clear or relevant. Overlooked populations have included people living in rural communities, people of color, women, men who have sex with men but who do not consider themselves gay, teenagers, and heterosexuals who have more than one sexual partner.

AIDS prevention programs have not targeted active and recovering alcoholics or others who use alcohol. There are, however, important areas of HIV-related risk for users of alcohol, and it is essential that these individuals receive HIV education and counseling.

Most providers and program planners who work with active and recovering alcoholics are in an excellent position to see that relevant, effective HIV education and counseling is provided. But without information about the links between alcohol use and the risk of HIV infection, it is impossible to give this issue the attention it requires.

Are There People with HIV Disease in Recovery?

Yes. People with HIV disease are participating in alcohol recovery. While there are few surveys investigating HIV disease in recovery programs, anecdotal reports indicate that alcohol recovery settings include both HIV-infected people and people with HIV-related concerns.

How Do Alcoholics Get HIV Disease?

Alcoholics get HIV disease in the same ways that other people do, but there are some factors specific to alcohol use that increase the risks for alcoholics to become infected.

Increased HIV-related risk behaviors. When people are mildly drunk, they become disinhibited, and they are less likely to follow some of the rules they normally would. A person who has made a firm commitment never to use injection drugs may change his or her mind when drinking. Someone who has sworn to use condoms and latex barriers during sex may "forget" or find it difficult to use them after a couple of drinks.

In fact, researchers have looked at the reasons why people who have followed safer sex practices for a period of time will slip and have unsafe sex. Alcohol is the single most commonly used substance associated with these slips in sexual behavior.

Blackouts. A common symptom of alcoholism is the "blackout." An alcoholic can swear to never having used injection drugs in one sentence, and in the next admit to having forgotten half the things he or she has done in the past 10 years. In a community of drinkers and drug users, it would be easy for someone to try injection drugs and share needles while in a blackout, and not to remember the event later. This makes it difficult for alcoholics to assess their risk of HIV infection and to prevent transmission to sexual and needle sharing partners.

Biological susceptibility. Laboratory studies have suggested a variety of possible effects which might increase susceptibility to HIV infection. In one study, alcohol impaired the responses of white blood cells to HIV. These important disease-fighting cells of the immune system help prevent or fight infection. In another study, a single episode of drinking limited the immune response of white blood cells, making these cells more susceptible to HIV infection.[1] A person using alcohol may actually facilitate the process of HIV infection by making it easier for the virus to establish itself during an unsafe encounter.

Polydrug use. Many alcoholics are polydrug users. While alcohol may be their drug of choice, many users have tried other substances including heroin, cocaine, or speed, all of which can be injected. People who have used injection drugs have usually shared needles at some point in time and this puts them at especially high risk of HIV infection.

Prevalence of HIV disease among gay-identified men. A large number of gay-identified men have become HIV infected through unsafe sexual contact. It appears that gay men also have a higher rate of alcoholism than of most other segments of society. The result is that gay men, some of whom are HIV-infected, are participating in recovery programs.

HIV can infect anyone. HIV infection is caused by a virus. The virus does not care if a person is gay, bisexual or heterosexual; male or female; old or young; Black, White, Latino, or Asian. Anyone who has unsafe sex or who shares injection equipment can become infected with HIV if his or her partners are HIV-infected.[1] (See also Appendix D: *Participant Training Tools* for a list of safe and unsafe sexual activities and instructions for proper cleaning of injection drug works.) People in recovery can be infected with HIV if they have been sexually active in relationships with men or women, one person or many, or because they have shared needles or injection equipment, one time or many times.

What are the Future Risks for People in Recovery?

There are also potential risks for people who are currently in recovery and who are not infected with HIV.

Relapse. Not all participants will succeed in a given effort to achieve sobriety. While this does not mean they cannot succeed in a future effort, it does mean that many people "go out" and start drinking again. Among participants who have used drugs, some will also begin to inject drugs and share needles again upon alcohol relapse.

New sexual relationships. Most programs advise participants in early recovery to avoid new romantic or sexual relationships. Nonetheless, some participants do become sexually involved with someone in the recovery community, someone who is still using, or someone—gay or heterosexual—who has had sexual partners in the past. Any of these individuals could be HIV infected.

Many people in recovery have not yet developed the self-esteem necessary to attend to their own needs or assert their desires. It can be difficult for a newly sober person to set forth his or her wishes, take steps to care for him or herself, and follow safer sex guidelines.

People who have been in recovery for a longer period of time also enter into new sexual relationships. The desire to be sexually close to another human being is a natural one, and it is something that many people anticipate as they grow in their recovery.

Involvement in already-established sexual relationships. Some participants come into recovery already involved in sexual relationships. Their partners may also be in the recovery community, may still be using alcohol or drugs, or may have had past sexual partners.

What Issues Arise When Providers or Participants Have HIV Disease?

In established recovery programs, such as recovery homes or outpatient clinics, there are some common issues that arise when providers or participants are known to have HIV disease.

Fear of infection. Some participants and providers are afraid of "catching" HIV disease from an individual who has the infection. HIV, however, is not transmitted through casual contact. The virus cannot pass from one person to another unless there is an exchange of blood, semen or vaginal secretions. Such exchanges can easily be avoided in day-to-day contact between recovery providers and participants.

Discrimination. Participants and providers may discriminate against people with HIV disease. They may believe that HIV-infected people will not benefit from a recovery program or that people with this life-threatening illness should not take up space in programs with limited resources.

Additionally, a disproportionate number of people with HIV disease are gay men, people of color, or poor people. When participants and providers interact with HIV-infected people, they may come face to face with old feelings of homophobia, racism, and classism. At a more subtle level, they may simply feel uncomfortable with someone they perceive as different from themselves.

In the past, recovery programs and providers have not limited care for people facing life-threatening illnesses. Individuals with cancer, liver disease, or heart trouble have not been excluded from services. People of many different backgrounds and experience have joined in and contributed to the recovery community. Similarly, people with HIV disease deserve to be welcomed and supported in the process of recovery.

INFECTION CONTROL. Participants and providers may not be familiar with proper infection control procedures. In residential, inpatient, or day-treatment programs, outpatient clinics, and private households, however, certain guidelines should be followed for the protection of all participants. People with HIV disease are susceptible to a variety of infections that would not affect someone with a healthy immune system. It is also possible, though much less likely, that a person who is not HIV infected could be exposed to HIV if he or she handles blood improperly during a first aid situation.

Finally, there are infections other than HIV—such as hepatitis B—that can pose a danger or cause inconvenience to anyone, and the transmission of many of these can also be prevented by proper infection control. Extensive "household studies" have found no instances of HIV transmission among people with family or housemates with HIV disease, except where specific risk behaviors, such as unprotected sexual intercourse or needle sharing, have occurred. (See also Chapter 4: *Facts about HIV Disease.*)

Recovery programs generally have legal obligations to follow infection control guidelines, and could be liable if participants become ill because the program has not taken proper precautions. (See also Appendix C: *Infection Control.*)

PHYSICAL ABILITIES. Some people with HIV disease have medical conditions that limit their level of physical activity. A participant may have difficulty, for example, doing housecleaning chores shared by members of a residential community or waking up in time for an early morning group. Providers will need to know how to properly assess such a situation. Is a participant's behavior a sign of physical illness, a symptom of resistance, or a form of acting out?

Each possibility must be carefully considered. Discussions with co-workers, a more experienced colleague, or the participant's medical providers can offer further insight in such a situation. (There are laws concerning the confidentiality of medical information and HIV-related information. Prior to discussions with others, providers will have to obtain HIV-specific releases signed by the participants in question. See also Chapter 7: *Legal Issues for Providers.)*

Alienation. Ignorance about the causes, course, and treatment of HIV disease can lead to suffering among HIV-infected people. For example, characterizing HIV disease as a death sentence, a hopeless situation, or something a person brought upon him or herself can contribute to a sense of alienation, despair, or hopelessness for a person with HIV infection. Providers and participants who are educated about the cause and course of HIV disease are less likely to have these beliefs or to make such statements.

Processing Feelings about AIDS. Programs, providers, and participants will need to deal with the feelings raised by serious illness, loss, and death. While this has not been a traditional feature of recovery programs, when providers or participants have HIV disease (or cancer, liver disease, or other life-threatening conditions), it is necessary to discuss such matters. Programs can implement activities that encourage the open expression and exploration of such feelings. Providers will benefit from trainings or consultations that help them improve their skills for facilitating such discussions in both group and one-to-one sessions. (See also Appendix D: *Participant Training Tools* for training information regarding grief and loss.)

What Should Recovery Providers Do?

When they were drinking, most participants did not make the best choices for themselves, their families, or their communities. In sobriety, particularly during early recovery, any kind of decision-making process is often difficult and confusing. People need help learning how to gather information, judge its reliability, and make healthy and positive choices. Many participants will look to providers to learn these skills.

To support these needs, recovery providers are encouraged to take three important steps:

Educate yourself, colleagues, and participants. All providers and participants need to be educated about HIV disease—what HIV is, how to prevent its transmission, and why people who use or have used alcohol have special risks for contracting it. This means that providers need to be able to talk comfortably about HIV infection, health, and sexuality with program participants.

Know about the HIV antibody test. Some participants will be interested in taking the HIV antibody test to find out if they are infected with HIV. Providers can help participants think about the decision to test or not to test. To do this effectively, providers must understand what the HIV antibody test is, what it does and does not tell people, and how people react to taking the test and hearing test results, especially during early sobriety.

Support people with HIV disease in the recovery community. People who have HIV infection will continue to seek recovery services and be active in the recovery community. Providers and administrators need to understand how the presence of HIV-infected people will affect program planning. Providers will want to know how other participants will react to the knowledge that there are HIV positive people in their programs, support groups, or other activities.

To offer the best possible support, providers must also be familiar with the special issues facing HIV-infected people in early recovery. Common issues are likely to include concerns about inclusion or exclusion within the program or community—"Do I belong to this group? Do I want to? Do they want me?"; apprehensions about changes in appearance, physical disability, or death; questions about whether recovery efforts are worthwhile in the face of another life-threatening disease; and confusion about just where to focus when dealing with the dual diseases of alcoholism and HIV infection. Administrators should establish policies concerning medical treatment of people with HIV disease, and consider what their program's response will be if an HIV-infected participant becomes seriously ill.

What about the Alcoholic Who is Still Using?

Active alcoholics also need information about their risks for HIV infection and how to protect themselves from HIV transmission. The presence of HIV infection, or the fear of becoming infected, often inspires a person to evaluate his or her life. The fear that one's life span might be shortened by HIV infection can create a tremendous crisis. In many cases, a positive HIV antibody test result or an AIDS diagnosis *is* the crisis—the bottom—that motivates a person to enter recovery.

While users may deny HIV-related risks associated with alcohol, it is important for providers to acknowledge that simply seeking information about HIV disease is an active step in self care and a positive and healthy choice. Providers can help alcohol users understand this and encourage them to continue making healthy choices in the future. These choices include decreasing or eliminating risks for HIV infection, and seeking further assessment or treatment for alcohol-related problems.

Wherever possible, providers should keep the door open for further contact with alcohol users. In the future, an active alcoholic may want more information about HIV disease, the relationship between HIV infection and alcohol, or his or her own drinking behaviors. Each contact can be another opportunity to educate a person about HIV prevention and another opportunity to urge the person to get help for alcoholism.

In terms of HIV prevention, providers can encourage active users to protect themselves from HIV disease, even if drinking and other drug use continue. Recovery is always a possibility, even for alcoholics far progressed in their disease. But once a person is HIV infected, alcohol recovery will not save him or her from the progression of HIV disease.

What about the "Social" Drinker?

There are some people who are able to drink socially and who are not alcoholics. But the disinhibiting effects of alcohol may be present even for a person who has had only one or two drinks. People unaccustomed to drinking may find these effects even more powerful. Add this to a situation where a person is feeling a strong sexual attraction, and the result may be unsafe sexual contact. Providers offering HIV prevention education can discuss the association between drinking and HIV transmission risks with all participants and clients, no matter how often they currently drink.

While the quantity of alcohol a person drinks is important in assessing alcoholic behavior, their pattern of drinking and the reasons for and consequences of their drinking is also relevant. If occasional drinking is associated with life-threatening behaviors—such as having unprotected sexual intercourse with a person who may be HIV-infected— it may be considered addictive drinking and, therefore, may require recovery intervention.

What's the Connection?

The connection between HIV disease and alcohol is not as straightforward as that between HIV disease and injection drug use or unprotected sexual intercourse. No unsafe "body fluids" are exchanged during drinking, so many people assume alcohol has no connection to HIV disease. It usually takes repeated education to convince drinkers and recovering alcoholics that they may face genuine HIV-related risks and that HIV infection is an issue of concern to them.

But the connection is clear. Alcohol can weaken the immune system's ability to fight infection. Alcohol disinhibits people and makes it more likely that they will participate in risky behaviors even if they have resolved to avoid unsafe sex and needle sharing.

Providers can help people see the important relationships between drinking behaviors and HIV risk behaviors. They can encourage participants to explore their own feelings about the epidemic, to consider their own past or present risks for HIV infection, and to evaluate their response to the presence of people with HIV disease in a recovery program. Providers can welcome participants with HIV infection and take steps to make the recovery setting a supportive and safe place for them.

Open and direct information about HIV disease and alcohol, paired with a foundation of compassion and understanding for all participants, will strengthen the ability of individuals to achieve and maintain sobriety. The HIV prevention message has the potential to save lives. By making this important effort to educate participants and colleagues about the connections between HIV infection and alcohol, providers offer an essential contribution to their programs and to the larger recovery community.

References

1. National Institute on Alcohol Abuse and Alcoholism. Alcohol and AIDS. *Alcohol Alert.* No. 15 (January 1992): 1-3.

CHAPTER TWO

LIVING WITH HIV DISEASE IN RECOVERY

In This Chapter:

- Jerry's Story: One Alcoholic's Experience
- HIV and Alcoholism: Similar Challenges
- Twelve Steps for People with HIV Disease
- Supporting People with HIV Disease

CHAPTER TWO

LIVING WITH HIV DISEASE IN RECOVERY

Jerry's Story: One Alcoholic's Experience

My name is Jerry, and I'm a recovering addict and alcoholic. I'm also infected with HIV, the virus that causes AIDS. My story is not a story about despair, or death, or the loss of hope. Instead it is about learning to live, about life, and most of all about recovery—recovery from my addictions, and recovery from my HIV infection.

In 1935, Alcoholics Anonymous was formed by two men. Two men who had tried every cure known to mankind for their chronic alcoholism. Men who had been told that if they continued drinking they would die. Men who had been told that they could not be helped. Men who had been told that there was something morally wrong with them because they drank. These men discovered that while they would never be cured of their alcoholism, they could recover. One day at a time, they learned that they could live with their disease.

I will never be cured of my alcoholism and addictions, but one day at a time I can be healed and one day at a time I can live my life to the fullest. This is the same way I live with HIV infection. I have learned that healing is very different from cure, and I have been able to heal so much in my life. I did not come to this understanding or acceptance overnight. It took many days of fear, struggle, denial, guilt, shame, terror and screaming at God, and that is the story I want to share with you.

There are a thousand and one similarities for me between being an alcoholic and being HIV infected. Both are diseases characterized by denial, guilt, fear, ignorance and shame. Both are diseases believed by many to be caused by moral failure: if you're an alcoholic, it's your fault. if you're HIV infected, it's your fault. Both diseases are believed to be incurable. When I discovered I was HIV infected, my life changed in ways it had not changed since I had first admitted I was an addict and needed help.

Fear and shame are all I remember from the first few days after I found out I was infected. This was not supposed to happen to me. I had been in recovery for four years. Sure, sure I had unsafe sex a couple of times. But it couldn't be possible that it had led to this.

No, no, no! I'm not ready to die!

Suddenly, I was dirty. Suddenly, I could not trust my body. Somewhere inside was a virus that was slowly killing me. Watching friends die of AIDS, I knew how painful and ugly that death could be. I did not know what to do.

For weeks I could not share the news with my friends. What would they think? What would they say? How could I have let myself become infected? Most importantly to me, how could they love me now that I was HIV infected?

Slowly, ever so slowly, I began to ask for help, to learn that I would not die tomorrow, that there were steps I could take, that there was hope.

The lessons of my recovery in AA were the tools I used to face my HIV infection. Once upon a time in my life I could see no other way to live but with drugs. At that time I was frightened, lonely, in tremendous pain, and I did not know how to be honest with other people or with myself. At that time my life seemed completely hopeless. I was now at a point where my life felt hopeless once more. I turned to what I knew. The Twelve Steps. I remembered, and realized again, that only after I accept things as they are, can I then take the action to change them. I learned again that while I can't change the reality of my being infected, I can choose between running the disease or having it run me.

I began to take action. I asked my friends for support. I sought out professionals who could help me make decisions about treatment. I educated myself. I no longer felt so powerless in the face of my infection. With the help of others I learned that I could stay healthy, one day at a time. Each day now I am grateful for my continuing health, and my continuing recovery. Each day I rediscover I am full of hope and full of life. Many days are difficult. Friends die, I feel tired, and I wonder. Many days I wish I could completely forget about HIV and AIDS. But I can't—just as I cannot forget I'm an alcoholic.

It has been four years since I first heard these words: "Your test result came back positive. Do you understand what a positive test means?" Four years of learning about acceptance, about faith, about death, and, most importantly, about living. I am blessed with good health, and I do everything in my power to ensure that I remain healthy. I do not know what the future will hold for me. I could someday get sick. I could someday pick up a drug or a drink. But this is no longer what I focus on. I focus on living. Now. Today.

So often I have heard a still-using addict or alcoholic say, "What's the use? I'm HIV infected, why should I stop using? I'm going to die, I might as well die using." That statement is filled with so much pain, so much fear, so much misunderstanding. Through the Twelve Steps, I have been shown a way of life that allows me to laugh, to hope, to love, to live life with a joy and a peace I never thought was possible. What a gift this is as I face the potential development of a life-threatening illness. I can live with this disease, just as one day at a time, I live with another disease in my life. After all, what other choice do I really have?

– Recovering Alcoholic with HIV disease

Jerry's story is about using the Twelve Steps to change his attitude toward a life-threatening disease. Most HIV specialists believe attitude plays a role in how people physically respond to HIV infection. It has long been known that some people do better than others when diagnosed with serious illness.[1] In many cases, the people who do well are committed to a cause or a belief, or have a sense of special purpose in their lives. They are likely to have good friends or close family—people whom they love and who love them. They may do volunteer or professional work they enjoy. They may express themselves artistically, through music or writing or dance, or have hobbies or pastimes that they find rewarding.

Attitude is not the only factor that affects how a person responds physically to a disease. But a person with the qualities listed above is likely to do better than a person who has no sense of purpose, no friends, and no hope.

HIV and Alcoholism: Similar Challenges

HIV and alcoholism have some similarities that are immediately obvious. Both are progressive, life-threatening diseases. Both can lead to premature death. Neither has a cure.

But there are other similarities that are also notable. Foremost is the great degree to which people misunderstand HIV infection. There is a lot of ignorance about HIV disease and, as with alcoholism, this ignorance can cause suffering. For example, many people think HIV infection is the result of moral weakness or bad acts. Some believe it is God's punishment of people who have sinned. They may say that people with HIV disease are to blame for having the disease.

Similar statements have been made about alcoholism.

Some people with HIV disease believe these statements and feel ashamed or guilty about being infected. They may think that they are evil, sinful, or worthless. They may believe they should be able to control the illness, and that if it progresses it is their fault.

Many alcoholics also feel this way about their alcoholism.

People with HIV disease sometimes choose not to tell friends, co-workers, landlords, or insurance companies about their infection. Letting people know can lead to lost friendships, job dismissals, evictions from apartments, or denial of insurance coverage. People may be afraid to seek treatment for HIV infection because they do not want records of treatment available to insurance companies or employers.

Alcoholics have made similar choices about treating the disease of alcoholism.

There are wonderful, caring nurses, doctors, and counselors who have reached out and helped people with HIV disease. But there are others who do not want to work with these individuals, people who are afraid that they will become infected with HIV from a patient or client, people who complain that they "don't like to work with those kind of people." Some have argued that people with HIV should not receive intensive and costly medical treatments because they are "hopeless cases."

Many alcoholics have had similar experiences with the health care community.

Alcoholism is a disease characterized strongly by denial—denial of the scope of the problem, denial of the effects of drinking, denial of the pain experienced by alcoholics and their families. People often approach HIV disease with considerable denial as well. Some people deny that they could be at risk for infection and avoid taking steps to protect themselves. Thoughts like the following support their denial:

- "Heterosexuals aren't really at risk for HIV infection, so I don't need to use a condom."
- "I only share needles with good friends, so I don't need to clean my works with bleach."
- "Sex with this man would be so exciting! It will be okay if I don't use a condom just this one time."
- "She looks so nice. I'm sure I don't have to worry about HIV with someone like her."

People may also use denial when they think about past behaviors that might have exposed them to HIV.

- "I'm just a lucky guy. This kind of thing wouldn't happen to me."
- "I've only had sex with six people in the last three years. That's nothing. I'm not at risk."
- "If something like that had happened to me, I would have known about it somehow. I don't need to worry."

Or people may tell themselves they do not need to consider taking the HIV antibody test (which indicates if a person is HIV infected). "Even if I was infected," they say, "there is nothing to be done about it." (See also Appendix B: *HIV Antibody Testing.*)

Denial about the real dangers of a disease can lead a person to engage in risky behaviors. For the alcoholic denying alcoholism, this might be trying to engage in controlled "social" drinking. For a sexually-active person denying the risk of HIV transmission, this might be having sexual intercourse without using a condom.

In both cases, denial can discourage people from seeking treatment for their illness. For the alcoholic, this might mean skipping AA meetings: "I don't need that any more; I've heard all that AA has to offer." A person with HIV disease might avoid seeing a physician or other medical provider: "I'm not feeling sick; there's no reason for me to see a doctor about any of this." But the group support provided by AA can keep an alcoholic from progressing in his or her disease. And medical evaluation and treatment, especially very early in the course of HIV disease, can help an HIV-infected person live a longer, healthier life.

These are some of the ways the hardships of HIV disease are similar to difficulties faced by alcoholics. But there is another way these diseases have proven similar: in the spiritual realm.

Most people working in the recovery field have heard others describe their gratitude for being an alcoholic. For many, the trial they face in confronting alcoholism actually strengthens them. They may learn new ways of loving themselves and others. They may develop a new relationship with a higher power. They may discover a new serenity in their lives.

There are individuals with HIV disease who have had similar experiences. Some, it is true, have felt hopeless and bitter about having the disease. But others, especially those who have been supported by family and community, have found a great spiritual serenity. Being told they had HIV disease was a life-transforming experience. The life they might have taken for granted before, suddenly became precious beyond all measure.

Alcohol recovery providers, familiar with the pain and isolation alcoholics suffer, can feel empathy for many of the experiences of people with HIV disease. This is a special insight that can be called upon when working with HIV-infected people. When wondering, "What is this person's experience? What is he or she asking for? How can I help?"—think back on the experience of working with alcoholics. There is probably something there that can guide you.

Twelve Steps for People with HIV Disease

Many people who are already familiar with 12-step philosophy have adapted these ideas for living with HIV disease. In some places, 12-step groups specifically addressing HIV have been established. Different versions of the Twelve Steps of Alcoholics Anonymous have been adapted for use at such meetings.

The 12-step philosophy works well for many people with HIV disease. The steps teach them to accept and face reality, and take responsibility for their own actions. The steps suggest people place trust in a higher power. This relationship with a higher power can help people in their efforts to make positive decisions for themselves and their communities.

The AA slogan "Awareness, Acceptance and Action" is an excellent guide for people with HIV disease. When they become aware of their infection, and then accept the reality of having this disease, they can take productive steps to promote physical and spiritual health.

People in recovery who have HIV disease may want to attend HIV-related 12-step meetings. Local AIDS information hot lines may know whether such groups have been organized and where and when they meet.

These groups will not be available in all areas. And some people who are committed to traditional interpretations of the Twelve Steps may not be satisfied with the adaptations that tend to be made at HIV-focused 12-step meetings. For example, in one adaptation, Step 2 reads, "Came to believe that a Power greater than ourselves could restore our peace of mind."[2] A suggested format for an HIV-Anonymous meeting includes, as part of the *Welcome*, a three-minute visualization of "healing light" entering and surrounding one's body, followed by the Serenity Prayer.[3]

Even if 12-step HIV groups are not available, or clients are not happy with the format of existing groups, the Twelve Steps can be applied on an individual basis to a person's issues about HIV disease. The steps contain a wisdom that is broad enough to address anyone's problems—whether it is being upset that a favorite football team lost the championship or discovering that one is HIV infected. One of the benefits of 12-step philosophy is its relevance to different people and situations.

Supporting People with HIV Disease

People with HIV disease are living in the recovery community. They are gay, and they are straight. They are former injection drug users, and they are people who never used needles in their lives. They are alcoholics who had blackouts and who don't know how they could have become infected. They are women and men who traded unsafe sex for alcohol or drugs. They are people who received blood transfusions after injuries or during surgery.* They are among the small number of health professionals who have become infected after suffering an accidental needlestick on the job. In the most important ways, they are no different from people who do not have HIV disease.

You might have met a person meeting one of these descriptions. But you might not know it if you did.

Ask at your own agency or program whether people with HIV disease would feel safe talking to staff or participants about HIV infection. Most of the time, people believe their organizations are supportive places in which people would feel fine talking openly about anything, including HIV infection.

However, there are many instances when participants choose not to tell others about their HIV infection. "I'll be rejected and become an outcast," or "They'll ask me to leave the program, or they'll make it hard for me to stay." Even staff members say, "I am HIV infected myself and do not feel it would be safe for me to tell my co-workers about it."

It is essential—the absolute foundation of AA—for alcoholics to share experience, strength, and hope with other alcoholics. Alcoholics who cannot share with others similarly afflicted do not have a very good chance of succeeding in recovery. The ability to

---

* Since 1985, blood donated for transfusions or other medical purposes has been screened for HIV infection, and blood infected with HIV is not used.

share experience and feelings is also important for people with HIV disease. Sharing leads to improved attitude and hope, which may actually help a person live longer and in better health.

For people struggling to stay sober in early recovery, knowing that there is support even if they have HIV infection may make the difference between success and failure in recovery. Recovery providers have always sought to create an atmosphere of openness and honesty in which participants can discuss and examine their recovery. By consciously considering the issues that face people with HIV disease in recovery, providers can ensure that the setting is accepting and encouraging for all participants. With this support, it is possible for HIV-infected alcoholics to achieve sobriety and serenity even in the face of such an uncertain and frightening disease.

References

1. Justice B. *Who Gets Sick: Thinking and Health.* Houston: Peak Press, 1987.
2. Hodge RH. 12 steps for coping with HIV infection. Montrose Counseling Center-Houston, n. d. Photocopied handout.
3. Mikluscak-Cooper C, Miller EE. *Living in Hope: A 12-Step Approach for Persons at Risk or Infected with HIV.* Berkeley: Celestial Arts, 1991.

CHAPTER THREE

THE LESSONS OF HISTORY

In This Chapter:

- The Early Years: Fear, Controversy and Confusion
- The Middle Eighties: Continued Resistance and Denial
- The Later Eighties into the Nineties: Slowly People Start to Come Around
- Coming in the Future. . .
- High Rates among People of Color
- The Lessons of History

CHAPTER THREE

THE LESSONS OF HISTORY

The history of the AIDS epidemic in the U.S. holds many lessons for the recovery community today. There was denial, confusion, and fear in the earliest years of the epidemic, which made it difficult for many people to see their true risks or to take actions to protect themselves from infection. Today, we have an opportunity to learn from past mistakes, as well as past successes, and to save lives by doing so.

The Early Years: Fear, Controversy and Confusion

In the early eighties, I offered an AIDS training to a group of mental health professionals working in a jail setting. Some of these providers already knew a lot about AIDS—they worked with a pretty high risk population and had had some experience with people who had AIDS. Others really wanted to learn more, both for their own sake and to help the inmates they worked with.

But one part of this group wanted to have nothing to do with the training. When I asked why, a psychologist said, "Oh, this whole AIDS thing just irritates me so much! Sometimes I wish all the gay men and drug users would just hurry up and get AIDS and die. Then we wouldn't have to worry about it any more."

– AIDS Educator

In the earliest years of the AIDS epidemic, from 1981 to 1982, scientists were baffled by this unusual disease that affected young, apparently healthy gay men. Doctors struggled, without success, to find effective treatments for their patients. People with AIDS kept getting sicker, and many of them died. The numbers of new cases continued to grow at an alarming rate.

There was a terrible fear in the gay community at this time. Gay men wondered who among their friends would be the next to become ill. They worried about causes and desperately sought ways to protect themselves. It was many months before it became evident that AIDS was being passed between sexual partners. Even then, it was not clear what specific activities were risky. No one was thinking that this disease was caused by a virus that might be in a person's body for five or 10 years before symptoms appeared.

Controversy developed as gay men and their doctors in the worst hit areas—San Francisco, New York, and Los Angeles—debated what to do to halt the epidemic. Some people advocated total sexual abstinence for gay men. Others suggested having sex with fewer people, or only with well-known friends or partners. A few promoted the use of condoms. And some felt these efforts to limit the open expression of gay sexuality were an affront to the hard-won freedoms of gay pride and gay rights, and were based on anti-sex feelings and not on scientific fact. Proponents of these differing points of view argued, and the debate added further confusion and turmoil in an already frightened community.

The bottom line was that people were being asked to change sexual behaviors. But changing these very personal and powerful behaviors, without clear guidelines on just what changes would be useful, was extremely difficult. With all the controversy, it was easier for many people to reassure themselves that their own risk was small and that behavior change was not necessary.

At this time, people outside the gay community were also being affected by AIDS. A number of Haitian immigrants in the U.S. and injection drug users, male and female, had been diagnosed. It was not always clear how or why these people had gotten AIDS—what their risks had been. Fear and confusion grew in these communities as well.

People hearing news reports about AIDS in the early 1980s learned that its causes were mysterious, its effects often disfiguring, its course usually fatal, and its cure or treatment unknown. Gay men were believed to be especially susceptible because many engaged in anal intercourse, which appeared to be particularly risky. Injection drug users were thought to pass the disease by sharing needles and other injection equipment. And Haitians were suspected, often inaccurately, of engaging in a variety of activities that might expose them to the disease, including male-to-male sex, ingesting blood in voodoo rites, and injecting vitamins and herbs with unsterilized needles.

As alarmed as people felt on hearing such reports, there was a certain reassurance among those who were not gay or bisexual men, not injection drug users, and not Haitian. "This is *their* problem," people seemed to say. "Since I don't do the things they do, I don't think this will affect me."

In the early 1980s, studies repeatedly demonstrated that the disease passed from person to person through sexual intercourse or blood-to-blood contact. Public education emphasized the fact that AIDS was not casually transmitted.

Despite these studies, people often felt a generalized fear of AIDS and addressed their fears by ostracizing those believed to be at risk. People in the so-called "risk groups" began to experience new episodes of discrimination. Haitians could not find jobs. Injection drug users could not find doctors. Gay men could not find apartments. Individuals believed to have AIDS were thrown off buses, removed from airplanes, or refused admittance to public schools.

The early years were characterized by ignorance and fear. Most Americans did not feel their own lives would be directly affected by AIDS. AIDS was a disease of urban, gay-identified men, a temporary issue that would not touch other people.

1981. . . A total of 227 cases of AIDS are reported. Of these, 85 percent are diagnosed in gay or bisexual men, and the majority are White men. One case in six is diagnosed in an injection drug user.

The Middle Eighties: Continued Resistance and Denial

In 1984, I was at a meeting of women who worked in AIDS services. One woman showed us an article from a medical journal. It described several children who were thought to have AIDS. All of them had a mother or father who had AIDS or was at risk for AIDS.

Many of us argued about this article. "There are a lot of diseases that would damage a newborn's immune system," we said. "We don't even really know what AIDS is. How can anyone say that infants have a disease that has only been seen in adults?"

This was naive of us. I know that now. But we really wanted to believe this disease was different; that somehow it was a disease that only affected one group, or a few groups of people.

– Social Worker

By the middle 1980s, the routes of transmission of HIV were well understood. It was known that HIV could be passed between individuals who exchanged blood, semen, or vaginal secretions. It was also known that a pregnant woman with HIV disease had a risk of passing the virus on to her fetus. Cases of male-to-female and female-to-male transmission had been documented in the scientific literature as well as in the popular press.

Nonetheless, there continued to be tremendous resistance to this information. AIDS was first introduced to the American public as a disease of gay men, and it was difficult for people who were not gay men to consider themselves at risk. Even among AIDS educators and providers, it was sometimes hard to see AIDS for what it really was: a disease caused by a virus to which anyone might be susceptible.

In 1984, this virus was identified. An international committee of researchers named it "HIV," human immunodeficiency virus. By the end of the year, a test to detect HIV antibody was developed, and it was in widespread use by March 1985.

The antibody test provided the means to identify HIV-infected people, even before they developed symptoms of illness. It became possible to screen blood donations for HIV and prevent transmission of the virus in blood transfusions. Anyone who wondered whether he or she had been infected could take this simple blood test to find out.

Even with the antibody test, many questions remained. If someone was infected with HIV, would he or she inevitably progress to AIDS? Could people rid themselves of HIV infection? Could doctors offer any help for people who tested positive? If not, was there really any reason to take the test in the first place?

At the beginning of 1985, more than 4,000 people in the U.S. had been diagnosed with AIDS. Still most did not feel touched in a personal way by the epidemic. The President had never uttered the word "AIDS" in a public speech or press conference. The sense of urgency experienced by members and friends of the gay community seemed absent in governmental settings. Press coverage focused on the sensational aspects of this "gay disease" rather than on its medical effects and rapid spread. Why, AIDS providers wondered, wasn't the country more concerned?

The actuality of heterosexual transmission—from men to women, and from women to men—had also been well-established by this time. The mysterious HIV-related risks in the Haitian community had finally been attributed, in large part, to heterosexual transmission. But it was difficult for the public to fully accept this possibility. Articles appeared in magazines and newspapers about the "myth" of heterosexual AIDS. Sexually active heterosexuals were confused by conflicting information. It was difficult to know what to do. Most did not change their behaviors.

Meanwhile, in the gay male community, sexual behaviors had undergone a significant change. Gay men were tending to have sex with fewer partners, using condoms for anal intercourse, and avoiding HIV-related risk activities. These behavior changes represented the most extraordinary changes in health behaviors ever seen in a population at risk for a health hazard—at levels far greater than had ever been achieved in smoking cessation, heart-attack risk reduction, or seat belt compliance efforts.

Why were gay men able to make these changes when others were not? Probably the single most powerful influence for those who made behavior change was knowing someone who had been diagnosed with AIDS. By the mid-1980s, most gay men knew someone with the disease; many knew someone who had died of it. AIDS was real to them, and it happened to real people they knew.

The diagnosis and death of one well-known public figure in 1985 helped change the American perspective on AIDS. Rock Hudson, robust and healthy idol of the heterosexual Hollywood dream, appeared gaunt and grim in news reports. He was said to be suffering from AIDS. After a brief period of sensationalistic press coverage and a flight to Paris in search of treatment, Hudson died.

Now, for the first time since the epidemic had started, most Americans "knew" someone who had had AIDS. There was shock and disbelief for many; Rock Hudson, widely perceived to be a virile heterosexual man, had contracted AIDS and died. There was also an outpouring of grief at his death. And there was a public acknowledgment that, while Rock Hudson's death drew much attention, thousands of Americans had already died of AIDS unnoticed by most of the country.

1985. . . 4,079 cases of AIDS are reported. The cumulative total since the beginning of the epidemic is 8,661. One in eight cases is diagnosed in a woman. A small number of cases, less than 2 percent, is diagnosed in a child. Fifty-nine percent of reported cases are among Whites; 25 percent among Blacks; 14 percent among Latinos. Among pediatric cases, nearly 80 percent are Black or Latino.

Fifty-seven percent of cases came from one of five major cities: New York, San Francisco, Newark, Miami, and Los Angeles. One in six cases continues to be diagnosed among injection drug users.

The Later Eighties into the Nineties: Slowly People Start to Come Around

In 1989 I took a night class on Contemporary Health Issues, and someone came to class to lecture about AIDS. I was a little anxious, looking back on it now, when instead of just lecturing, the guy had us get involved in a "Time Line of HIV Disease." He put this big time line on the wall. It ran from 1980 to the future , and each of us had to write when we first heard of AIDS; when we first knew someone—friend, family member or co-worker—with AIDS; and when, if ever, we had been involved in an AIDS-related job or volunteer work.

I was amazed where my classmates fit on this time line. It was a real spread. Some folks knew about AIDS for years before I ever even knew it existed. Some folks remembered hearing about it on TV early on in the epidemic, and other folks found out about it when their friends died. It was kind of heavy; actually, it was really heavy.

The clincher came after we'd had some time to look at the things we'd written and talked about. The instructor had us answer the question, " When did you first think about your own risk for AIDS?" My first thought was that I never have , and I didn't need to. But when we got to talking, it was a revelation. Suddenly all these risky situations I'd been in over the years surfaced: people I'd been with—I mean, slept with—drinking, taking drugs. All of it was risky, and at the time, I hadn't thought twice about it.

What an eye opener! I had to admit, to myself anyway, that there were a lot of situations in the past, maybe in the present, that I couldn't be sure about.

– Student in Alcohol Studies Program

By the late 1980s, more people in the U.S. were beginning to understand that this massive epidemic would touch most people in some way. In 1989, the U.S. cumulative case load reached over 100,000. In 1990 alone, nearly 40,000 cases were reported. This was no longer a disease that affected strangers in far away cities. Neighbors and friends, co-workers, and children and parents were being diagnosed. All kinds of people, from all walks of life, found themselves infected by an accident of coincidence combined with some HIV-related risk.

In the mid- to late eighties, treatments for HIV disease finally became available. Antiviral medications slowed the progression of the disease for many people, and special treatments were sometimes able to prevent the occurrence of *Pneumocystis carinii* pneumonia, the leading cause of death among people with AIDS. People with HIV infection began to live longer, healthier lives.

In October 1987, the Names Project Quilt was laid out in front of the Capitol Building in Washington, D.C. This powerful display brought together quilt panels memorializing thousands of people who had died of AIDS. In its subsequent national tour, millions of people who viewed the quilt witnessed the loss of this epidemic in a powerful way. The quilt panels, carefully constructed, so personal in nature, named friends and lovers, uncles, brothers, children and mothers who had died of AIDS. It was so much more possible to see that each name, each number in the growing toll, was a person with a life, with friends and family, with love and pain.

In late 1991, another well-known public figure acknowledged being infected with HIV. Magic Johnson, one of the finest athletes in the country, a man widely-respected and deeply loved by fans, tested antibody positive. A few months later, Arthur Ashe, the well-known tennis player, also announced that he was HIV-infected. Once again, the public was stunned to see in action what HIV educators had been saying for years: "Anyone can get HIV disease. Male or female, black, brown or white, gay or straight, famous or unknown, weak or strong." This disease is caused by a virus. The virus doesn't care who you are.

It has taken a full decade, but now many people know that HIV infection is a fact of modern life. People are beginning to understand that anyone can contract the disease if exposed to the virus. They are much more likely to believe that HIV disease might be a risk for them personally.

Unfortunately, there is still a long way to go before people really follow through on HIV prevention guidelines. While it is known precisely what activities transmit the virus and that avoiding these activities can prevent transmission, new infections continue to occur every day.

1991. . . 45,000 cases of AIDS are reported. The cumulative total since the beginning of the epidemic is over 200,000 cases. Among all cases to date, about two out of seven have been diagnosed among injection drug users. Because of the additional cases of AIDS among sexual partners and children of injection drug users, one out of three cases can be traced to injection drug use.

African-Americans and Latinos continue to be diagnosed in numbers greater than their proportions of the total population would suggest. About three out of 10 cases are reported among African Americans; about one out of six is reported among Latinos. More than 20,000 women have been diagnosed with AIDS, as have over 8,000 teenagers and young adults under age 25.

Coming in the Future. . .

I often ask people if they've ever had a sexually transmitted disease. If they have, I ask them if they were drinking when they got it. And I'll ask them if the person they got it from was drinking when he or she got it. It's really unusual not to find alcohol somewhere in the loop. Somebody was drinking somewhere, slipped a little around sex, and—boom—you got the clap.

HIV is no different. Except symptoms of the clap show up in a couple of weeks, and symptoms of HIV may not show up for five or 10 years. And the clap can usually be treated with antibiotics while HIV, a disease that can be fatal, has no cure.

This is why it's really important for people to protect themselves every time they have sex. And we need to remember that drinking interferes with a person's reasonable ability to do that.

– Alcohol and Drug Counselor

There is no question that HIV disease will be with us for a long time. Clues gathered by scientists today offer some ideas about where the epidemic is heading in the future. Some of the trends are relevant for alcoholics, both active and in recovery.

It appears, for example, that injection drug users and their sexual partners are continuing to be infected with HIV at disturbing rates. While some users are cleaning needles, many do not do so every time. And it has been difficult to persuade some injectors to use condoms during sexual intercourse. These circumstances are of special concern for alcoholics who use or have used injection drugs, or who have had sexual partners who have used injection drugs.

There are also studies showing that young gay men and gay men of color are more likely to engage in unsafe sex. Many believe HIV infection is a disease afflicting gay White men in their thirties and forties. Some younger gay men feel they are not in danger as long as they choose other young partners; men of color may consider themselves free of HIV-related risk if they have sex with other men of color. Among young gay men or gay men of color, who participate in recovery programs, there are likely to be individuals with significant HIV-related risk histories.

Recent surveys of sexual behavior among gay men have shown a trend to "relapse" in sexual behaviors. Men who have been following safer sex guidelines for several years have slipped on one or more occasions and had unsafe sex. The use of alcohol has been strongly associated with this kind of relapse behavior. It is likely that the association of alcohol use and sexual relapse is common across different population groups.

Alcoholics in early recovery may feel overwhelmed by the perceived complexities of sex in sobriety. When approaching sexual situations, the thought of discussing or practicing safer sex can further increase their discomfort. The appeal of old and familiar behaviors, in relation both to drinking and sexual practices, may be heightened in these "slippery" circumstances.

Meanwhile, denial contributes to the practice of unsafe behaviors among women and men of all sexual orientations. Denial is a defense mechanism necessary to sustain alcoholic behavior. Alcoholics in recovery tend to use denial because it is a particularly familiar defense. It is easy for someone who customarily uses denial, consciously or unconsciously, to deny the severity of HIV-related risks. In such a frame of mind, the practice of unsafe behaviors can easily be rationalized.

These trends suggest some likely outcomes for the future spread of HIV infection:

- The numbers of gay men with new infections will probably decline overall. However, men who have sex with men will continue to be infected, especially men in their twenties and teens, and men of color.
- Injection drug users will continue to be infected. In communities with intensive, ongoing education about cleaning needles, their numbers may be lower. Free needle exchange programs—by which a person can exchange a used needle for a new, sterile one—are also likely to lower the rate of new infections.

- Heterosexual women and men will continue to be infected through unsafe sexual contact with injection drug users or other HIV-infected individuals. The numbers will remain smaller than the number of gay men or injection drug users infected. However, the actual proportion of heterosexual cases may increase over the next several years. In 1991, about 8 percent of cases involved heterosexual transmission. In the future, this percentage may be higher.
- People of color, especially African Americans and Latinos, will continue to be diagnosed with AIDS in numbers higher than their proportion in the total population.

High Rates among People of Color

At the beginning of the epidemic, little energy or money was given toward HIV prevention education in communities of color. The disease continued to be viewed by most of the public as a disease of gay White men long after scientists and policy makers knew this was not the case.

Additionally, economic and social situations have contributed for a long time to health problems among poor people and people of color in this country. Federal, state, and local governments have made few resources available to promote health and prevent illness among poor communities. When people do become ill, they often have nowhere to go for medical care. There are few resources available for alcohol recovery or chemical dependency treatment.

Warnings from the federal government or other "outsiders" have carried little weight in communities that have been neglected, lied to, and maltreated in the past. HIV prevention messages produced with the mainstream, dominant culture in mind have little relevance for people who are strongly identified with different cultures. When local people are not given the resources to provide HIV prevention education themselves, compliance with prevention guidelines is likely to be limited.

These are the circumstances under which a disease like AIDS can easily take hold, spread, and grow. This explains, at least in part, the higher rate of HIV disease among African Americans and Latinos.

The Lessons of History

In the mid-1980s, I worked for a project doing AIDS prevention for teenagers. At the time, there were only a few teens in the whole country who had AIDS, so it was hard to convince anyone that teenagers were at risk.

Sometimes, we had a hard time convincing ourselves. We worked with young people out on the streets. They lived hard lives. They prostituted, dealt and used drugs, had lots of unsafe sex and shared needles. But we didn't see them getting AIDS. We didn't know then that it could take five or 10 years for symptoms to show up.

We made up reasons for the low rate of AIDS among these teens. "Teenagers have a different kind of immune system from adults, so they don't get infected," we said. Or, "They need to go through many years of unsafe behaviors before they could possibly get AIDS. It can't happen to them when they're this young." Or even, "These kids are lucky to be alive, given what they've gone through. They're survivors. They won't get it." Sounds like denial, doesn't it?

A couple weeks ago, I met a 20 year old woman who has HIV disease. She was 13 and out on the streets of this town when I first started doing AIDS prevention work. She was prostituting and having unsafe sex with her drug-using boyfriend. This is almost certainly the time at which she was infected.

I don't think I knew her then. But if I had, I wonder if I could have really believed in her risk. I wonder if I could have convinced her. Because I had my own denial about it, I'm not sure I was as persuasive as I might have been. Or could be today, when I know that there are probably over 200 teenagers with HIV infection here in my community.

We really need to believe in the risks of this disease, and communicate this to people in a direct, personal, and emphatic way. This is as important for alcoholics and people in the recovery community today as it was for that teenager seven years ago. I hope we don't make the same mistakes now that some of us made then. We have all the evidence we need—HIV is out there, it's real, and it's a danger. We have got to let people know that.

– HIV Educator

What the history of the HIV epidemic shows, over and over again, is that no one wants to be at risk for HIV disease. Early on, people wanted to see AIDS as a disease of gay men, or of Haitians, or of drug users. They did not want to see it as a human disease that might affect anyone.

As a culture and as individuals, we often use denial to minimize our own perception of HIV-related risk. We comfort ourselves with the thought that HIV disease strikes people who have had "a lot of sexual partners," even though people who have had only one sexual partner have become infected. We think it is a risk for people who inject drugs daily with any stranger they meet, not for someone who shot a little speed with friends a few years back. We use this sense of denial to rationalize current behaviors—not using a condom, for instance, because, "This person just doesn't seem like someone at risk for HIV."

Finally, and sadly, we have learned that HIV continues to act as viruses do, infecting new individuals when any opportunity arises. Our denial has proven to be a poor weapon against HIV. In the early years of the epidemic, gay men did not have the privilege that everyone else has today: they did not know what behaviors put them at risk for HIV disease. Our current knowledge about HIV transmission and prevention is a tremendous gift. Now it is up to us to use that gift to protect ourselves, and to encourage others in the recovery community—including our clients and participants—to protect themselves as well.

CHAPTER FOUR

FACTS ABOUT HIV DISEASE

In This Chapter:

- Answering HIV-Related Questions
- "AIDS" and "HIV"
- HIV Transmission
- Who Gets HIV Disease
- HIV Prevention
- Detecting HIV
- The "Spectrum" of HIV disease
- HIV-Related Treatments
- Special Issues for Women
- Pregnancy
- Special Issues for Children
- Living with HIV disease
- HIV and Alcohol: Important Connections
- Recovery and HIV Disease
- Follow-Up Information

CHAPTER FOUR

FACTS ABOUT HIV DISEASE

Answering HIV-Related Questions

The women who come to our program face many issues. They are alcoholics or addicts, or they are children or partners of alcoholics and addicts. Sometimes they are all of these people.

They are poor; they don't know where they'll be living or how they will feed themselves or their kids. Their lives have been filled with instability, uncertainty and gross violence. And most of them haven't even begun to deal with their own alcoholism or other addictions, so you begin to wonder where HIV fits in.

Once they're in the shelter, some women do see their alcohol addiction as an immediate problem, as something they need to deal with. They're ready to accept help to stop drinking and begin recovery. Other women don't see the problem, and don't want help. But we always talk about alcoholism and addiction, we always offer interventions, and we never give up the message.

We had to work as a full staff to get clear about how to deal with the AIDS crisis for the women in our program. And we realized that it was really important for them to have the information. So we deal with HIV the same way we do with the message about addiction: we talk about it with everyone, and we never give up the message.

It helped for us to get good information for ourselves, and simple answers to a lot of our own questions about HIV.

– Staff Person at a Shelter for Battered Women

Participants will have questions about HIV disease and AIDS if providers give them the opportunity to ask. To respond accurately and supportively to their questions and concerns, providers need some basic information about HIV disease. It is important for providers to know the information, and have straightforward, clear answers to share with participants. This chapter provides answers to common questions about HIV infection.

Information about HIV disease appears to change all the time. TV programs, magazines and newspapers often describe new scientific reports or other information. However, the most important facts that can help stop the spread of the virus have not changed: these include how HIV is transmitted and how people can prevent transmission.

People with HIV-related concerns deserve to be treated with dignity and respect, no matter what they ask. A person may have HIV infection, have a friend or family member who is infected, or be afraid of becoming infected. Whatever the issue, when people feel respected, their true concerns are more likely to come forth, even if these concerns are embarrassing or confusing. When people do not feel respected, they are likely to withhold important questions. It is useful to keep this in mind when answering participants' questions about HIV disease and AIDS.

"AIDS" and "HIV"

What is AIDS? What is HIV?

AIDS stands for "acquired immunodeficiency syndrome." It is a life-threatening disease of the human immune system. People with AIDS are likely to get a number of diseases that do not affect people with healthy immune systems.

HIV is the name of the virus that causes AIDS. HIV stands for "human immunodeficiency virus."

In most cases, a person infected with HIV will live for many years without becoming seriously ill, often without any long-lasting symptoms of illness.* Eventually, mild signs or symptoms of immune system problems do develop and gradually worsen. When

---

* It is important to note that during this "asymptomatic" phase, people with HIV disease can transmit the virus to other people.

damage to the immune system has progressed considerably, it usually leads to serious illness, which is often indicated by an AIDS diagnosis. This evolution is known as the spectrum of HIV infection.

HIV-infected people are said to have HIV disease. While many people use "HIV disease" and "AIDS" to mean the same thing, it is important to note that HIV disease refers to the whole spectrum of HIV infection, and AIDS refers to a specific set of serious medical conditions that result from HIV infection. These conditions are usually the most life-threatening HIV-related illnesses.

Where did AIDS start?

Scientists believe that HIV originated in Africa, probably as the result of the natural mutation of another virus. This is the accepted scientific response.

There are other people, however, who have different beliefs about the origins of HIV, despite the fact that there is no evidence to support these beliefs. For example, some believe HIV was the result of biological warfare research—an experiment gone awry. Others consider HIV to be a deliberate attempt at genocide, seeking to wipe out gay people, injection drug users, and people of color. Still others theorize that HIV is the result of a biological accident involving contamination of medicines or vaccines.

Whatever its source, HIV disease is now a worldwide problem that is affecting all races, both genders, all classes, and all types of people. The entire world must collaborate to stop the spread of the disease.

HIV Transmission

How do people get infected with HIV?

HIV has been found in a number of different body fluids including: blood; any body fluid containing visible blood; semen; vaginal secretions; menstrual blood; and human breast milk. There are additional internal fluids surrounding organs, joints, or membranes that carry HIV. Health care workers need to take precautions in situations when open sores or cuts may come into contact with these fluids, but other people are unlikely to be exposed to them.

People usually become infected with HIV by taking the blood, semen or vaginal secretion of an infected person into their own body. There are four typical ways this might happen.

UNPROTECTED SEXUAL INTERCOURSE. People can exchange blood, semen, or vaginal secretions through unprotected vaginal, anal, or oral intercourse. "Unprotected" means without the use of a condom or other latex barrier. Semen used for donor insemination for women attempting pregnancy can also transmit HIV.

SHARING OF NEEDLES OR OTHER INJECTION DRUG USE EQUIPMENT. When people share needles or works for injection drug use, they are also sharing small quantities of blood. HIV can be present in that blood. Sharing needles for tattooing, ear or body piercing, injecting steroids or insulin, or other purposes is also dangerous.

FROM AN INFECTED WOMAN TO HER FETUS OR NEWBORN. A pregnant woman who has HIV infection may pass the virus on to her fetus or newborn. There is an approximately 20 to 25 percent chance that the child of an infected woman will have HIV. There are three ways such infection might occur: a fetus may be infected during the course of pregnancy; a newborn may be infected during the birth process; or a baby may be infected by feeding on the breast milk of an HIV-infected woman.

EXCHANGE OF BLOOD, TISSUE, OR OTHER INTERNAL BODY FLUID. Early on in the AIDS epidemic, a number of people were infected with HIV through blood transfusions. Some people with hemophilia who were treated with medicines manufactured with human blood were also infected. Medicines for people with hemophilia are now manufactured so they are free of HIV. Since 1985, blood donations have been tested for HIV, and transfusion-associated HIV infection is extremely rare today.

A few individuals have become infected with HIV after receiving body tissue or organ donations from a person with HIV disease. Tissue and organs are now tested before being used in human transplants.

Health care workers may be exposed to the blood or internal body fluids of patients, and some health care workers have become infected with HIV through accidental needlesticks or other mishaps. Health care workers are urged to follow universal infection control precautions to avoid the transmission of all blood-borne diseases, including HIV infection. These guidelines have been established by medical experts and, when followed regularly, can prevent infection of health care workers in most instances. (See also Appendix C: *Infection Control.*)

HIV is not transmitted through casual, day-to-day contact with family or friends. People do not need to worry about contact with tears, saliva, sweat, sputum, vomit, feces or urine, unless visible blood is present and their skin is broken and comes into contact with the fluid.

Can people get HIV infection from oral sex?

Yes. There are some well-documented cases of HIV transmission through oral sex. Most cases of transmission caused by oral sex involve the swallowing of semen. However, there are individuals who have been infected by HIV whose only acknowledged risk factor is having oral sex performed on them by a person with HIV. Transmission seems most likely to occur if one partner has mouth sores or bleeding gums, but these need not be visible.

Vaginal secretions and menstrual blood also carry HIV, and it is believed that HIV could be passed to a person performing oral sex on a woman with HIV.

Can people get HIV infection from just one unsafe encounter?

While repeated exposure to the virus obviously increases the chances of becoming infected, there are cases of people who have become infected after having only one, or only a few, encounters with a person with HIV disease.

Can people get HIV infection from insect bites?

No. There has never been a documented case of HIV passed from insect to human and no other data supports this possibility.

Epidemiologic studies (studies of who gets HIV disease, and how and where they get it) emphasize the fact that HIV is not passed through insect bites. Consistently, throughout the world, people diagnosed with HIV or AIDS are those who have engaged in some risk-related activity, such as unprotected sexual intercourse or the sharing of injection drug equipment. Children, who often receive the highest number of insect bites in a community, are rarely diagnosed with HIV infection, and only where another identifiable risk exists, for example, having received an HIV-infected blood transfusion, or being born to a mother with HIV disease.

Additionally, household studies of people with HIV disease have shown transmission occurs within a household only when identifiable risk activities have taken place, for example, from a man to a woman who have had unprotected sexual intercourse. Household members who presumably might have been bitten by the same insects have not developed HIV infection.

Do condoms really work?
Can they keep you from getting HIV infected?

Condoms do work in preventing the transmission of HIV. But they do not work 100 percent of the time.

Experienced condom users have much lower rates of condom failure (breakage or slipping off during use) than people who are not experienced.[1] Condom users can gain familiarity and comfort by practicing use of condoms in non-sexual situations. (See also Appendix D: *Participant Training Tools* for a training on condoms and latex barriers, and illustrated descriptions of proper condom and latex dam use.)

What methods for cleaning needles really work?

The best method for avoiding the transmission of HIV through needle use is never to share needles or works. If it is necessary to share, flush needles, syringes, spoons, or any other equipment with bleach before sharing. (See also Appendix D: *Participant Training Tools* for illustrated instructions on proper needle cleaning.)

Is it dangerous to live with someone who has HIV disease?

No. A few simple household cleaning routines will keep a house safe for the person with HIV and anyone who does not have HIV. (See Appendix C: *Infection Control* for a full description of infection precautions in residential settings. These guidelines are applicable in private homes as well as in organized residential programs.)

I hear a lot isn't known about HIV infection. How can we be sure that HIV is not casually transmitted?

Actually, quite a bit is known about HIV infection. The ways in which HIV can be passed from one person to another are well-established, as are methods to avoid such transmission. The presence of HIV infection can be detected in individuals carrying the virus. A number of treatments are now available which improve the outlook for HIV-infected people.

What is not known today is how to stop the progression of HIV disease once someone has the infection. HIV infection cannot be cured at this time.

Well-tested scientific methods have been used to examine HIV transmission, and studies of thousands of individuals reinforce the same information: HIV is not transmitted through casual, day-to-day contact.[2] HIV infection can only be established if the blood, semen, or vaginal secretions (or one of several internal body fluids or tissue) of an infected person enters someone else's body.

The incubation period for AIDS can last 10 years or more. How can we be sure that there aren't many people infected through casual contact who are now in that incubation period?

It may take 10 years or more from the time a person is first infected with HIV to the time when he or she is actually diagnosed with AIDS. Antibodies to HIV, however, develop in a fairly short period of time—usually two weeks to six months after infection. The HIV antibody test, which measures the presence of HIV antibody in the blood, can tell with considerable accuracy whether a person is HIV-infected. This means that if someone were infected through casual contact, there would be measurable evidence of this within a short period of time.

Studies that have looked for evidence of casual transmission have examined household contacts among families where an individual has HIV disease and residential school settings where students are known to have HIV. Dozens of such studies have been carried out. Every study of this nature ever performed has found absolutely no evidence of casual transmission.

About 3 percent of AIDS cases in the U.S. have an "undetermined" risk factor. How did these several thousand people get infected? Couldn't they have gotten it through casual transmission?

There are currently over 200,000 cases of AIDS reported in the United States. Gathering data on so many individuals is a difficult task. It is not surprising that information is incomplete for some of these cases.

However, the Centers for Disease Control (CDC), a branch of the federal government that keeps statistics on the HIV epidemic, has looked at this question carefully. With follow-up questioning, most individuals reported as "no identified risk" are found to have well-established risk factors (sexual contact with an infected individual, or an individual suspected to be infected; or sharing of injection drug equipment). The reasons the CDC cannot establish risks for some individuals include the following:

- The most common risk factors for HIV infection—sharing injection drug equipment or having unsafe male-to-male sexual contact—involve highly stigmatized behaviors. Some people do not want to admit engaging in such activities.
- Some people visit a medical clinic when they are ill and do not return for later follow-up care. Blood may be drawn or other diagnostic tests may be run at that initial visit. The AIDS diagnosis may be established after this, but because the individuals do not return for follow-up, no further information on risk factors can be gathered.
- Some people are too ill at the time of diagnosis to provide information about risk factors.

- Some people are diagnosed with AIDS after they have died. Information about risk factors may be unavailable.
- In a very few instances, individuals who do not actually have AIDS have been inappropriately classified as AIDS cases. Refinements in the diagnosis of AIDS have made this an unlikely problem today.

Who Gets HIV Disease

Who can become infected with HIV?

Anyone who is exposed to HIV can become infected. This means that anyone who has unprotected sexual intercourse, or who shares needles or other injection drug equipment, can become infected if he or she engages in that behavior with someone who has HIV disease.

Are heterosexuals really at risk for HIV? How come most of the sexually transmitted cases of AIDS are among gay men?

In the United States today, most sexually transmitted cases of AIDS are found among gay men. The disease was first identified among gay men and, because gay men as a group tend to have more than one sexual partner, the virus spread quickly in that group.

The number of U.S. AIDS cases caused by heterosexual contact, however, is on the rise. In 1984, for example, heterosexual contact accounted for less than 1 percent of all U.S. AIDS cases—about 50 individuals. At the end of 1991, 8 percent of the cases were the result of heterosexual contact. By that time, about 12,000 people had contracted AIDS through male-female sex since the epidemic began. More than one in four of those cases was diagnosed in 1991 alone.

In many other countries, AIDS is primarily a disease of heterosexuals. The World Health Organization estimates that 10 million people worldwide were infected with HIV at the beginning of this decade. By the year 2000, they expect that figure to rise to more than 25 million, and the number of cases among women will

Adult/Adolescent AIDS Cases by Exposure Category

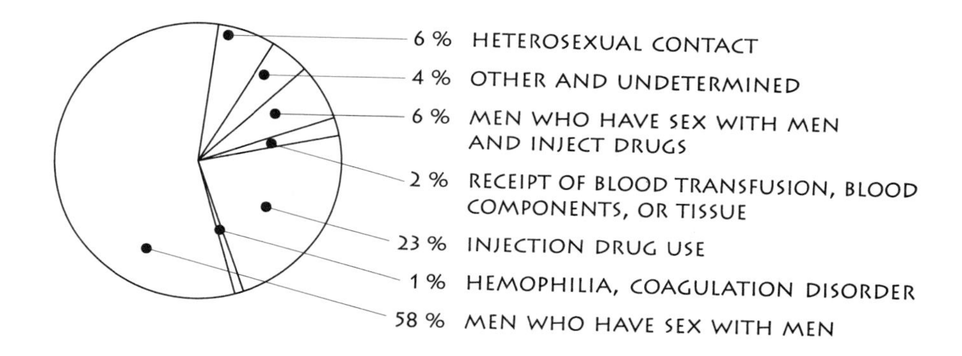

AIDS Cases by Race/Ethnicity

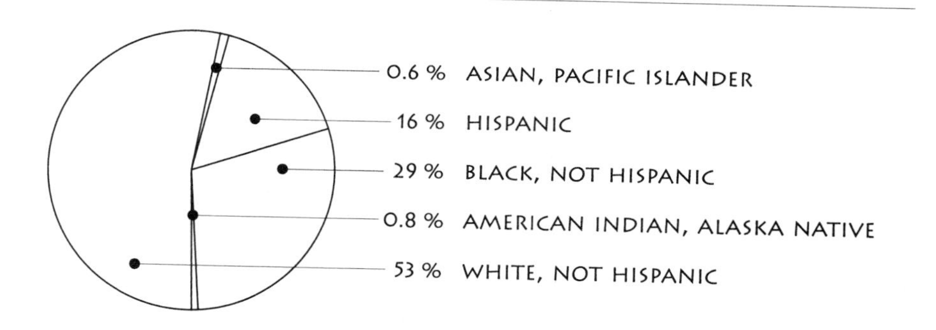

From Centers for Disease Control. *HIV/AIDS Surveillance Report*. April 1992.

approximately equal the number among men. Most of those infected will be heterosexuals.

Clearly, the HIV-related risks for heterosexuals are real and compelling. But, the relative risk for heterosexuals in most parts of the U.S. today is still low. The way to stay free of HIV infection is to follow safer sex guidelines and to avoid sharing needles.

Do lesbians get HIV disease? How?

Lesbians become infected with HIV the same way other people do: the blood, semen, or vaginal secretions of an HIV-infected person enters the body. This may happen through needle sharing, through unsafe sexual contact, or through an occupational exposure for a health care worker. Lesbians with HIV disease have not been especially visible because most reporting systems for HIV infection or AIDS lack categories identifying lesbians.

Lesbians who have sex only with women might engage in unsafe sexual activities that could expose them to HIV. Some lesbians have had sex with men at some point in their lives and may have been infected with HIV at that time. Others have used injection drugs and shared needles. Some have used donor insemination to conceive a pregnancy; if a woman's donor is HIV-infected, the woman is also at risk.

Can teenagers become infected with HIV?

Teenagers can become infected with HIV the same way anyone else can: taking the blood, semen or vaginal secretion of a person with HIV into their bodies. This might happen through unsafe sexual contact or the sharing of needles or works for injection drug use.

Teenagers with HIV disease have not been especially visible. Because a person can be HIV-infected for many years before showing symptoms of illness, many people infected as teenagers do not receive HIV-related diagnoses until they are in their early to mid-twenties and will not show signs of serious illness or be diagnosed with AIDS until later. At the end of 1991, over 8,000 people between 13 and 24 years old and 32,000 people 25 to 29 years old had been diagnosed with AIDS.

Teenagers, as a group, tend to have unsafe sexual contact with a number of different partners and to experiment with drugs and alcohol. Rates of sexually transmitted disease (STD) continue to be highest among teenagers and young adults. The potential for a teenager to become infected with HIV is real, and HIV prevention education for teenagers is extremely important.

Is HIV disease more of a problem in communities of color than in White communities?

The rate of HIV infection in communities of color, especially among African Americans and Latinos, is higher than their overall representation in the general population. African Americans account for about 12 percent of the U.S. population, but, to date, nearly 30 percent of AIDS diagnoses are among African Americans. Similarly, Latinos represent 9 percent of the U.S. population, but have been diagnosed with 16 percent of AIDS cases.

Health problems are usually more severe in communities that also suffer from poverty and inadequate education. At the outset of the HIV epidemic, most communities of color saw AIDS as a disease of gay White men, and AIDS education programs were not effective in disputing this myth. The federal government eventually warned people of color about AIDS, but these warnings carried little weight in communities that had been neglected or lied to in the past. All of these circumstances contribute to some degree to the higher rates of HIV infection in African-American and Latino communities.

In addition, treatment options for people of color are often limited by poverty, poor education, lack of insurance, and difficulties accessing services and care. People of color with HIV-related conditions are likely to receive poorer care, to suffer more episodes of severe illness, to be diagnosed later in the course of their illness, and to die sooner after that diagnosis than Whites. And poor people, whatever their ethnic background, are likely to have significant barriers to obtaining prevention information and to receiving HIV-related care if infected.

HIV Prevention

How can people protect themselves from HIV?

The two most important steps any individual can take to protect him or herself from HIV infection are:

- Do not have unprotected vaginal, anal, or oral intercourse with anyone unless you know that individual does not have HIV disease. Consider the limits to "knowledge" about people's sexual history and infection status. People who have engaged in an HIV-related risk activity can be infected without knowing it. In addition, people with sexually transmitted diseases, including HIV disease, have been known to lie to sexual partners about this, because they are eager to have sexual intercourse.
- Never share needles or other equipment for injection drug use or other purposes. If you must share, clean needles with bleach before sharing.

In addition, health care workers can lower their work-related risks by following universal infection control precautions for avoiding transmission of blood-borne diseases.

How can I encourage friends, colleagues, and participants to follow HIV prevention guidelines?

Research so far has pointed to one especially important influence on a person's choice to follow HIV prevention guidelines: the belief that their peers are doing likewise. Wherever possible, it will be helpful to reinforce any signs that peers—others in your friendship network, other colleagues, and other participants—are following prevention guidelines.

What is safer sex? What are examples of safer sex activities?

"Safer sex" (sometimes referred to as "safe sex") includes sexual activities that do not involve a high risk for HIV transmission. This means they are activities that carry little or no risk of exposing partners to each other's blood, semen, or vaginal secretions. Some examples of safer sex activities include:

- Mutual or solo masturbation.
- Massage, erotic touch.
- Reading or writing erotic stories; watching erotic films.
- Telephone sex (talking about sex on the phone with someone).
- Watching someone else touch themselves sexually.

(See also Appendix D: *Participant Training Tools* for a list of safe and unsafe sexual activities.)

What about kissing?

There has been some controversy about passionate, open-mouthed kissing. Kissing has never been shown to transmit HIV, and if there is any risk, it is apparently quite low. The theoretical risk comes not from HIV in saliva, but from the possible presence of infected blood in the mouth. A person with gum disease or sores in the mouth might bleed during passionate kissing. In very vigorous kissing, even a person with a healthy mouth might bleed. If the open gums or sores of one partner are exposed to the infected blood of the other partner, HIV transmission may occur.

What is a latex dam or barrier? How is it used for oral sex?

Latex dams are flat pieces of a thin rubber-like material, similar in texture to a condom, about six inches square, that are manufactured for use in certain kinds of dental work. They can isolate a section of the mouth and keep it dry. During mouth-to-vagina or mouth-to-anus sex, these flat pieces of latex can be used to prevent HIV transmission. The dam is placed over the vulva (women's genitals) or the anus (asshole), keeping fluids from being exchanged between sexual partners.

Dental dams are made of fairly thick latex, however, and many people feel the thickness limits the pleasant sensations of oral sex. Some people recommend "cutting down" a non-lubricated condom instead. After making a cut with scissors along one side of the condom, the thin latex can be placed flat over the vulva or anus.

People have also suggested using clear plastic wrap, or microwave wrap, as a barrier in oral sex. However, this thin wrap is easily torn. No scientific studies have looked at the effectiveness of any kind of flat barrier in HIV prevention. Studies have shown, however, that latex condoms can prevent HIV transmission and it is reasonable to believe a "cut down" condom, properly used, will also be effective. (See also Appendix D: *Participant Training Tools* for instructions on the use of latex barriers.)

If two people know each is HIV infected, is there any reason for them to practice safer sex together or to clean needles before sharing?

HIV mutates (changes its genetic structure) quickly. Because of this, there are a number of different strains of the virus. Some research has suggested that an individual infected with one strain of HIV who is subsequently infected with a different strain is likely to become seriously ill more quickly.

This means that a person with HIV disease, who has unsafe sex or shares needles with someone else with HIV disease, risks being infected with a different strain of the virus. There are individuals who have carried two or three different strains at the same time.

Additionally, a person with HIV who has unsafe sexual contact with another individual risks other sexually transmitted diseases, including herpes, venereal warts, hepatitis-B, syphilis, gonorrhea and chlamydia. Many of these diseases are particularly dangerous for HIV-infected people, and some can be life-threatening.

The best choice for maintaining health for people with HIV disease is for them to avoid unsafe sexual contact or needle sharing with another person, even if that person is also HIV-infected.

Detecting HIV

What is the HIV antibody test? What does it tell us?

The HIV antibody test is a simple blood test that indicates whether or not a person carries antibody to HIV, and, in this way, is the easiest way to determine whether someone is HIV-infected. The human immune system produces specific antibodies for each type of foreign substance, including HIV, that invades the body. If the antibody test result is "positive," it means antibody to HIV was found in a person's blood and he or she is HIV-infected and is capable of passing the virus to others.

If the antibody test result is "negative," it means no antibody to HIV was found. Either the person is not infected with HIV, or the person is infected with HIV and has not yet developed antibodies. It is important to note that it usually takes anywhere from two weeks to 12 weeks, and sometimes as long as six months, between the time a person is first infected to the time antibodies can be detected in the blood. On rare occasions, it may take longer. This period of time is referred to as the "window period."

How often should people take the test?

The answer to this question will depend on individual circumstances. A person's HIV antibody test result will be quite reliable as long as he or she is not tested during the window period. If the person's last possible exposure to HIV was more than six months ago, he or she would only need to take the test one time.

However, if a person has a negative test result (indicating that no HIV antibodies were detected), and the last possible exposure to HIV was three months ago, most counselors would recommend the person be tested again in three months to make sure the window period is fully covered.

Taking the test does not stop HIV infection. Stopping risk behavior does. Some people continue to engage in HIV-related risk behaviors, and repeat the antibody test regularly. Counselors working with these individuals will want to address the pattern of continued risk, and can use the test taking and counseling activity as part of a process to support a reduction in risk behaviors.

What are some of the reasons for someone in recovery to take, or not to take, the HIV antibody test?

People who take the antibody test and find they are negative (indicating that they are not infected with HIV) can benefit from the peace of mind this information gives them. They can make a commitment to avoid HIV-related risk behaviors in the future and thus maintain their negative HIV infection status.

People who take the test and receive a positive result (indicating that they are infected with HIV) can see a physician for evaluation of their immune system's functioning. Medications that can help people stay healthier and feel better are available at certain stages of HIV disease. In some cases, medical care for HIV infection, even in the absence of physical symptoms, can prevent the development of life-threatening illnesses. Additionally, people with HIV disease can make a commitment to avoid HIV-related risk behaviors, which can pass the infection on to others.

These are important benefits for anyone considering taking the antibody test. However, there are some potential drawbacks, especially for someone in early sobriety, which should also be considered.

The major concern is how newly sober individuals will emotionally handle the process and results of testing. People who take the test have to endure a lot of waiting—initially, a few days or weeks before the first testing appointment when blood is drawn, then another two weeks before the results become available. This waiting period can be a time of considerable tension for some people.

A person who tests negative on the antibody test, but is still in the window period—when infection may be developing—must wait an additional span of time before repeating the entire testing process and receiving a result in which he or she can have confidence. This can also be a stress filled process.

People usually have deep emotional responses to positive antibody test results. Those who test positive face a life-threatening and frightening illness. How well will people in recovery handle the anxiety associated with positive test results? Will they be able to continue making progress in recovery? Will they experience difficulty maintaining sobriety during this time?

In some instances, it may be better for a person who is still developing strength in his or her recovery, or for someone who is in crisis and in danger of relapse, to postpone decisions about testing. Someone who tests positive and reacts by giving up on a recovery effort is unlikely to acquire the medical care necessary to treat HIV disease, while again suffering the consequences of active alcoholism.

There are also more general concerns that anyone thinking about the test should consider. Primary among these is the matter of confidentiality: Is there any chance the test results could be shared with an insurance carrier? an employer? a landlord? others who the participant would prefer not know? (See also Appendix B: *HIV Antibody Testing.*)

Why is counseling such an important part of antibody testing?

People have many complex emotions and common misunderstandings about HIV disease and antibody testing. Before they can give proper informed consent to take the test, they must understand the risks and benefits of the test, the limitations of the test, and the actual procedure for testing. They should also have an opportunity to ask questions about HIV disease and antibody testing and have these answered. Pre-test counseling affords an opportunity for all of these needs to be addressed.

Post-test counseling—the session at which people receive antibody test results—is crucial in helping people respond to their test results. First, they must understand the meaning of the test result in terms of their current health. Second, they must evaluate their past risk history and current behaviors. Is there any chance they are still in the window period of infection? Are risk activities continuing? Do they understand fully how to prevent future transmission of HIV—either to themselves, if they are negative, or to others if they are positive?

People who test positive need to understand the value and importance of medical screening and care. They may need referral to an HIV-knowledgeable provider or to a low-cost medical clinic that can help them. They will want to think about disclosing their test results : who among their friends, family, and colleagues can support them, and who might present problems in reaction to disclosure? Perhaps most important of all, people who test positive will need help responding to the emotional ups and downs of a positive test result, along with referrals for support resources (for example, counseling and support groups) if appropriate.

All of this information must be relayed during the moments immediately after giving a test result, when clients are usually experiencing strong emotions: relief for people who test negative, uncertainty for people in the window period, and confusion, despair, fear, or shock, for people who test positive. Sometimes counselors are surprised by emotional responses: a person who tests positive may be relieved to have ended the uncertainty of whether he or she is infected; a person who tests negative may feel isolated among his or her friends, all of whom are HIV infected. Suicidal thoughts are not unusual among people who have just tested positive. Trained counselors can help clients cope with the emotional consequences of testing in a way that also allows time for sharing the important information that must be included in the post-test counseling session.

Should people in early recovery take the antibody test?

This is a complicated question. Providers and participants should evaluate this question on a case-by-case basis. (See also Appendix B: *HIV Antibody Testing.*)

The "Spectrum" of HIV Disease

What is the difference between "HIV infection," "ARC," and "AIDS"? What is "HIV disease"?

Anyone who has been infected with HIV, regardless of the state of his or her health, has "HIV infection" or "HIV disease."

"ARC" stands for "AIDS related complex." While this term was used earlier in the epidemic, it is rarely used today. People who had symptoms suggestive of AIDS, but who did not meet the government criteria for an AIDS diagnosis, were said to have ARC.

"AIDS" is diagnosed when a person with HIV infection meets one or more specific medical criteria as defined by the federal government. This might be the diagnosis of an HIV-associated infection, such as *Pneumocystis carinii* pneumonia; the appearance of HIV-related wasting syndrome, which involves profound weight loss without an identifiable cause other than HIV disease; or the development of HIV-related dementia (forgetfulness, inability to solve problems, difficulty thinking). Most often, whether or not severe symptoms are present, AIDS is diagnosed at an advanced stage of HIV infection, when the immune system is significantly weakened.

Spectrum of HIV Infection and HIV Disease

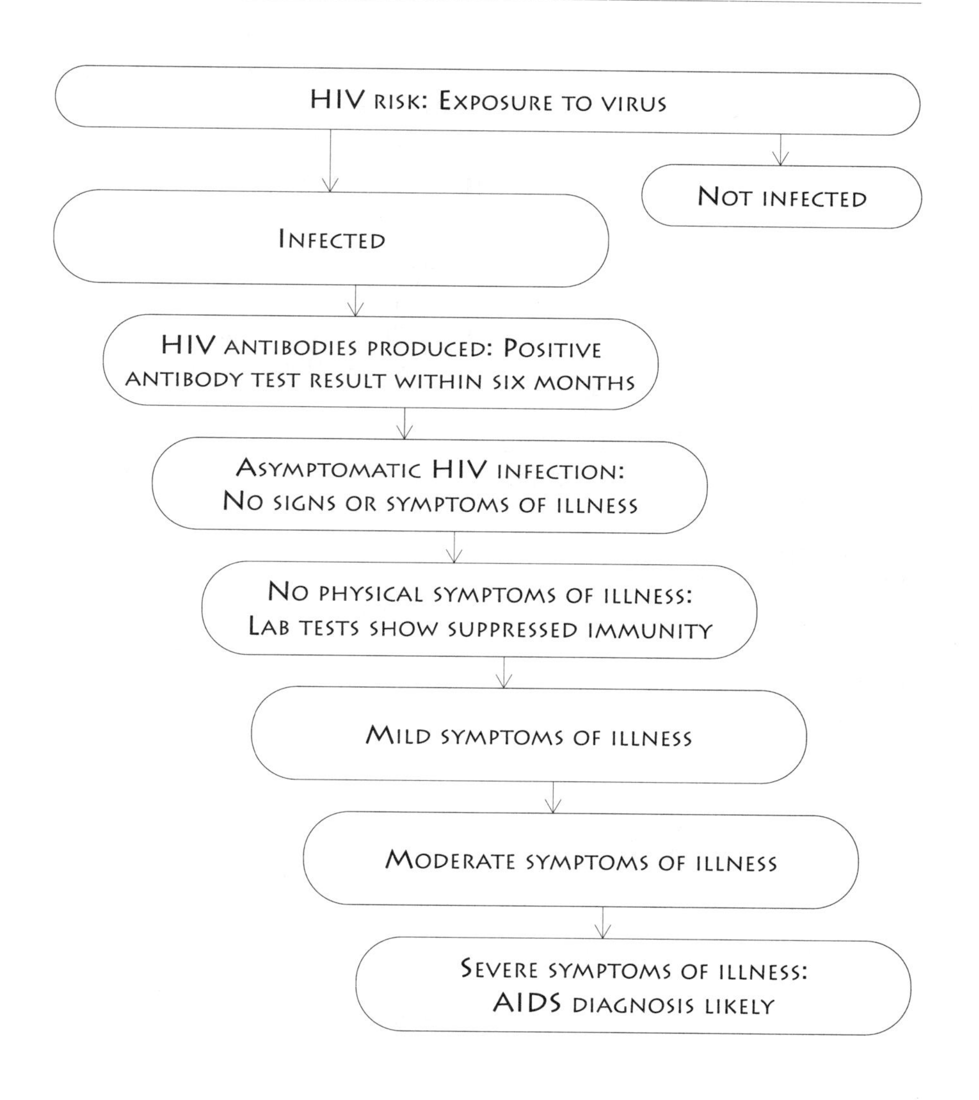

People with HIV infection may fall anywhere along the spectrum of disease. In general, HIV disease is progressive. People have no symptoms at the outset, but tend to develop symptoms over time. The rate of progression varies from person to person. After 10 years of infection, about half of those with HIV infection will have progressed to severe symptoms and an AIDS diagnosis.

HIV infection, then, spans a wide spectrum of medical conditions. Some people with HIV infection feel and look physically vigorous and healthy. Others have mild physical symptoms, such as fatigue, skin rashes, or occasional night sweats. Some have more serious, even disabling, medical conditions, and might qualify for an AIDS diagnosis. "HIV disease" is the most common term used to describe this range of HIV-related presentations.

How does HIV damage a person's immune system?

HIV affects many different cells of the human immune system. The virus can directly infect cells that play an essential role in protecting the body from disease. When a cell is infected with HIV, it is unable to act in the body's defense. The virus is able to take over the reproductive mechanisms of the cell to produce more viruses.

When a virus, bacteria, or toxin enters the body, a healthy immune system responds by identifying the intruder and manufacturing a specific defense against it. In a person with HIV infection, the body might not be able to identify the outside agent. If it does, it might not be able to manufacture the defense necessary to defend the body. If the special cells necessary for defense are manufactured, they may not operate properly and may not be able to help the body fight illness.

How long can a person be infected with HIV before progressing to an AIDS diagnosis?

Each person's response to HIV infection is different. Some people progress rapidly, others more slowly, in their disease. Most people with HIV disease will feel fairly healthy for an average of four to five years after becoming infected. After 10 years of infection, over half will have gone on to develop a severe HIV-related illness. However, there are individuals who have had HIV infection for 10 or 12 years, who still feel physically fit, and who are symptom-free.

I heard that the federal government is revising the definition of AIDS. What is the new definition? Why do they keep changing it?

The government had planned to change the definition of AIDS, but decided in June 1992 to indefinitely postpone this change. The new definition of AIDS would have added to the list of those conditions that qualify as "AIDS," certain laboratory guidelines, specifically the T-helper cell count, which shows if the immune system is seriously damaged (even when there are no symptoms of disease).

When AIDS was first described, in 1981, no one knew what caused the disease. Scientists with the federal government developed a "surveillance definition"—a definition that would allow them to see and count cases of the new disease. The definition was based on what the disease looked like among gay White men who had severe physical symptoms, because those were the cases that first came to the attention of doctors.

Since 1985, HIV antibody testing has made it possible to find out whether someone is infected with HIV. Further research and experience has shown that most HIV-infected people have no symptoms of illness; some have mild to moderate symptoms that do not qualify for an AIDS diagnosis; some have severe symptoms that are less common and therefore have not been included in the diagnostic guidelines for AIDS; and women, children, people of color, injection drug users, and poor people can have a number of HIV-related illnesses that are not included in the guidelines. The new diagnostic guidelines would have helped identify more people who have significant damage to their immune systems.

Is HIV disease a "death sentence"? Will everyone diagnosed with AIDS die of the disease?

HIV disease is serious, and an AIDS diagnosis is an indication that HIV infection has progressed to a life-threatening stage. Up to the present time, most people diagnosed with AIDS have survived less than two years. However, each person with HIV infection or AIDS is an individual, not a statistic. What is true for groups of people with HIV disease or AIDS—as expressed in statistical projections—is not necessarily true for every HIV-infected person. New research on treatments is proceeding rapidly. Doctors are hopeful that soon HIV disease will become a "manageable" condition, like diabetes or high blood pressure, and that with proper medication and monitoring, people will live a more normal life span.

Many people have lived well with HIV disease for years, and plan to do so for many years more. It is most useful to think of HIV disease as a life-threatening, rather than a fatal, illness. Describing HIV as a "death sentence" is misleading, and such statements can have a detrimental effect on the attitudes of people with HIV infection and others in the recovery community.

HIV-Related Treatments

How will an HIV vaccine work? When will it be developed?

Vaccines are currently under development, and some are already being tested. Vaccines are made from dead virus, parts of a virus, or synthesized viral parts. They mimic the virus and cause a person's immune system to respond by mounting a defense against the virus and the disease it causes, for example, the flu, measles, or polio. There are two kinds of HIV vaccines: those that seek to defend against a new infection of HIV, and those aimed at defending against the progression of an existing HIV infection. This second type works to improve the health of already infected people.

Vaccine development takes a long time, including periods of laboratory testing, animal testing, and a particularly long period of human testing. It is likely that it will be many years before a vaccine is widely used.

Prevention of infection by adopting safer behaviors is the only effective "vaccine" available today, and the only thing people can be sure of for the future.

What treatments are available for a person with HIV infection?

There is a wide range of medical treatment now available for people with HIV disease. These include antiviral medications that slow the progression of HIV disease, medications that help prevent occurrences of opportunistic infections, and treatments for the specific diseases and conditions that develop in HIV-infected people. Anyone infected with HIV is encouraged to see a knowledgeable medical provider to find out about these options.

There are also a number of alternative treatments, including acupuncture, herbal and Chinese medicine, homeopathy, vitamin therapy and visualization. Many people with HIV disease combine Western medical approaches with some of these alternatives.

People with HIV can take an active, decisive role in selecting a treatment option, or a combination of options, that seem most likely to help. For some people, however, access to treatment may be limited. This may be due to a number of factors including: limited financial resources to pay for expensive treatments: lack of information about options; geographic limitations, since new treatments may be available only to participants of medical studies, and these studies may be located only in some regions; or study eligibility requirements that may exclude women, children, injection drug users, and other categories of people.

What is "early intervention"?

Early intervention involves the use of diagnostic or treatment options early in the HIV disease process. Often, this includes taking action before physical symptoms of disease appear.

Early intervention includes HIV antibody testing to determine whether or not infection is actually present. For the person who does have HIV disease, early intervention involves immune system testing to measure the progression of disease, and development of a treatment plan consistent with test findings. The treatment plan might include standard Western medical approaches, alternative treatment options, involvement in HIV support groups, community activism, psychotherapy or counseling, or volunteer work. It might also involve treatment or recovery services for people with substance dependencies.

Special Issues for Women

What are the HIV-related risks for women?

The HIV-related risks for women are the same as those for anyone else: when the blood, semen, or vaginal secretions of a person infected with HIV are taken into the body, a woman can become infected. This might happen through unprotected sexual intercourse (vaginal, anal, or oral), or the sharing of needles or injection drug works.

Are symptoms of HIV different for women? Does the disease progress differently in women?

Most large-scale HIV-related studies have followed male subjects, and it has taken longer for studies of HIV disease and women to be pursued. Still, providers experienced with treating HIV infection in women have been able to draw some conclusions.

Women with HIV infection are likely to develop a number of gynecological signs of immune system suppression. Most common of these are vaginal yeast infections (candida) that are especially severe in nature and do not respond well to standard treatment. In the presence of HIV infection, sexually transmitted diseases may result in more severe gynecological symptoms, for example, herpes and genital warts. Women with HIV disease also appear to have a higher frequency of pelvic inflammatory disease (PID) than other women.

Statistics show that women do not live as long as men after a diagnosis of AIDS.[3] This is probably because women postpone medical treatment and are diagnosed later in the course of their illness, and because treatments that slow the progression of HIV infection have not been made easily available to women. Women, for example, have been excluded from many of the experimental protocols testing new HIV-related drugs.

In what other ways are HIV-related issues different for women than for men?

Women from all walks of life have been infected with HIV. As a generalization, however, women with HIV disease tend to be poor, undereducated, women of color, and mothers. For such women, it is difficult to locate and utilize health care and social support.

While most gay men have an easily identifiable community of support for HIV-related concerns, women with HIV disease usually feel isolated and alone. They may not know other women with HIV infection. They may be responsible for the care of children, and be accustomed to putting their own needs last. They may have little or no money, and no practical means of transportation to medical clinics or social services. They may be victims of domestic violence. They may suffer from depression, or be addicted to drugs or alcohol. Often, they are coping with a number of these complex issues in addition to illness, and this complicates access to treatment and care.

Medical and social services for people with HIV disease have often been developed to be accessible to gay men and responsive to their needs. Women with HIV infection may not feel included or comfortable in such programs. Practical material needs are often not met in these settings. For example, women themselves need toiletries, tampons, and sanitary napkins. Their children need diapers, and formula and other food suitable for children. If child care is not available, women may be unable to use these medical and social services.

Because the diagnostic criteria for AIDS have been based on common manifestations of severe HIV disease in men, women with severe HIV disease have not be diagnosed with AIDS. While they suffer significant disability, it has been difficult for them to qualify for certain free or low-cost financial and medical benefits and services without an AIDS diagnosis.

Pregnancy

What are the chances a pregnant woman with HIV disease will deliver a baby with HIV disease?

A pregnant woman with HIV disease has a 20 to 25 percent chance of delivering a child who is also HIV infected.

What should a pregnant woman do if she has HIV disease, or has a risk for HIV infection?

A pregnant woman with HIV infection needs to consider two important issues: the consequences of pregnancy for her overall health and state of mind; and the risks and consequences for her child should she choose to carry her pregnancy. While there are many options she can evaluate, the most basic is whether to carry or terminate the pregnancy.

Pregnancy does not appear to speed up the HIV disease process. However, it does create emotional and physical demands which can be challenging for any woman coping with a serious illness. A woman who already has moderately or severely symptomatic HIV disease may not wish to take on the additional demands of pregnancy.

A woman with HIV disease will want to think about the 20 to 25 percent chance that her child will also be infected with HIV. Most children born with HIV infection will have short lives complicated by severe and painful illnesses.

Additionally, a woman will want to consider the demands of childrearing. If she experiences an episode of illness, is there someone who can help with child care? If she becomes incapacitated or dies, is there an individual or family who can raise the child in a way she would like?

A pregnant woman who has been exposed to HIV-related risks should consider taking the HIV antibody test to determine whether she does, in fact, have HIV infection.

Ideally, a pregnant woman with or at risk for HIV disease would be able to discuss these issues and options with a trusted medical provider: a physician, a nurse practitioner, or a counselor. It is important for a woman to understand that the decision to carry or terminate pregnancy is her own. The advisor's role is to provide the information the woman needs to make an informed decision.

If she decides to continue her pregnancy, providers monitoring her pregnancy and delivery should know about her situation so they can provide the best possible care for her and her child.

Providers should remember that for many women, the ability to bear children is extremely valued. And for some women, a 75 to 80 percent chance of having a healthy baby does not seem like bad odds. Women with HIV disease must make their own choices about reproductive issues.

How can people ever plan pregnancies if they are always supposed to practice safer sex?

People who are confident they do not have HIV infection can safely conceive and carry pregnancies. There is no HIV-related risk associated with sexual intercourse or donor insemination if both partners are free of HIV infection.

If there is some question about past HIV-related risks, a couple planning a pregnancy could take HIV antibody tests to be sure each partner is free of infection.

Special Issues for Children

How do children get HIV disease?

The most common way for children to get HIV infection is perinatally—before or during birth, from an HIV-infected mother. Some children contract HIV during fetal development, the period when the fetus grows in the mother's uterus. Others apparently are infected during the birth process itself. In some cases, children have become infected through breast-feeding.

It is possible for a child to contract HIV sexually, if he or she were sexually molested by an HIV-infected person. A child suffering a needlestick from a recently discarded syringe might also be at risk. (HIV, however, does not live long or well outside the human body and is not easily transmitted through needlesticks.)

A small number of children (age 12 and below) are sexually active or experimenting with drugs. These children—if they share needles or practice unprotected intercourse—face the same HIV-related risks as adults. If the children drink during sexual activities, they may experience the same disinhibition effects as adults.

Is the HIV antibody test performed on children?

The HIV antibody test can be performed on children. Depending on state laws, a parent or guardian may be required to give consent for the test.

The antibody test is of limited use in newborns. For the first 12 to 15 months of life, a child carries some of its mother's antibodies in its blood. An HIV antibody test performed in this period may show positive results if the mother had HIV disease at the time of birth. The child's HIV antibody status cannot be confidently determined by this test until he or she is about 15 months old. Other experimental tests currently available may be useful in determining HIV infection in this newborn period.[4]

Are the symptoms of HIV disease different for children? Does the disease progress differently in children?

HIV disease tends to progress more quickly among children born with HIV infection than it does among adults. Most children will probably be quite ill by two years of age. There may, however, be a difference in the course of illness between the fetus infected during pregnancy and the newborn infected during delivery. While adults with HIV develop unusual illnesses that are not seen in people with healthy immune systems, infants and young children with HIV often develop severe cases of common childhood diseases. These illnesses tend to respond poorly to treatment.

The most typical problems for children with HIV include failure to thrive (poor growth and development), chronic diarrhea, bacterial pneumonia, and neurologic irregularities.

Unless the biological mother is known to be HIV infected, or children with HIV disease themselves become ill, infected children are unlikely to come to the attention of medical providers. There are recent studies which have found that some children born with HIV infection have done very well for many years. While most HIV-infected children have greatly shortened life spans complicated by serious illnesses, a few have lived to age 10 and beyond without serious health problems.

Living with HIV Disease

What is it like to have HIV infection? What is it like to have AIDS?

The experience of living with HIV infection and AIDS is different for everyone. Stage of infection and severity of immune system damage will affect a person's medical status and influence how he or she feels.

Some people with HIV disease look and feel healthy and vigorous. Others are often tired. Others suffer chronic, painful conditions. Still others feel they are on a roller coaster of medical ups and downs.

HIV disease is also characterized by emotional ups and downs. As the disease progresses, people often find themselves anticipating the loss of cherished capabilities: strength and energy, eyesight, wit and concentration, or physical attractiveness. It often seems that just as the person with HIV disease adjusts to one loss—"I no longer have the stamina to swim a mile, but I love swimming so I'm just settling for doing less,"— something new comes up—"The doctors think I have pneumonia again, and I can't walk more than a block without having to stop and catch my breath."

Parents of minor children must consider questions of child care and custody—"Who will take care of the children if I become seriously ill or am hospitalized? Who will raise them if I die?" People who look forward to the promised benefits of a new medication may find they are unable to tolerate the treatment. Friendships and primary relationships shift and change, sometimes growing stronger and at other times crumbling. All of those coping with this life-threatening disease contemplate their own death. Most can do this at some moments with equanimity, at others with fear and even panic.

How can attitude help people cope with HIV disease?

Mental attitude has a lot to do with how a person feels when coping with a serious illness. It is always difficult to adjust to a disease which saps strength, causes pain, and disfigures one's appearance. But a person who feels hopeless and has few resources and few friends is likely to have a much harder time with HIV disease than someone who has a strong spiritual program, a lot of hope, and a positive outlook on life. Good financial and personal resources, a healthy friendship network or community, and a sense of spiritual serenity can all contribute to a positive attitude and more successful coping styles.

HIV and Alcohol: Important Connections

What's the connection between alcohol use and HIV disease?

People who have as little alcohol as a single drink will experience some impairment of fine motor coordination and judgment. Many will also experience disinhibition—they find themselves doing things they would not do if they were not drinking.

This combination of effects means that people who have made a commitment to practice safer sex may not abide by that commitment if they have been drinking. They might feel it will not matter if they engage in some HIV-related risk, or they might judge that an activity is risk-free when it isn't. The clumsiness associated with drinking makes it difficult to use condoms or latex barriers. People are likely to find it easier to slip into risky behaviors after a couple of drinks. (See also Chapter 1: *HIV and Alcohol: What's the Connection?*)

Is there a connection between immune system damage by HIV infection and the damage caused by drinking and alcoholism?

Chronic use of alcohol damages the immune system in a number of well-documented ways:

- Chronic alcoholics have decreased white blood cell counts. As a result, the body does not respond to infections well.
- Alcohol-related liver disease damages the body's ability to produce T-helper cells, which are essential in fighting diseases. Chronic drinkers have low numbers of T-helper cells.
- Alcoholism is associated with the development of some cancers.
- Chronic alcohol abusers generally have poor nutrition. Their overall health suffers as a consequence.
- Alcohol use interferes with the body's ability to use vitamins and minerals properly. This leads to immune system damage.

Interestingly, HIV infection leads to some similar problems in the immune system. People with HIV disease often have low numbers of T-helper cells and nutritional problems, and HIV disease is associated with the development of certain cancers.

There is continuing debate, however, about whether the use of alcohol or other drugs has any effect on the progression of HIV disease. One study reported that HIV-infected people who used substances did not progress to AIDS any more quickly than those who did not.[5] Others have criticized the methods of this study and believe that alcohol or drug use does speed up the disease process.

Some researchers have suggested that the immune suppression caused by chronic alcoholism makes it easier for alcoholics to become infected when exposed to HIV. Until further information is available on these matters, it seems prudent for people with HIV infection to avoid all drugs, including alcohol, except those prescribed by a health care practitioner and used as directed. Individuals who use alcohol or other drugs are strongly urged to avoid using substances before or during sex because of the dangers associated with these combinations.

Recovery and HIV Disease

Can a person with HIV disease benefit from a recovery program?

Absolutely! Many people find the spiritual and practical tools of a 12-step recovery program to be of great help in learning to live with HIV disease. In fact, AA's Step 12 includes the phrase "tried to...practice these principles in all our affairs." (See also Chapter 2: *Living with HIV Disease in Recovery.*)

Is there a connection between co-dependency and HIV risks?

Co-dependency is a state where an individual consistently puts the needs of other people before his or her own to an extent that is physically or emotionally damaging. There are certainly some HIV-associated risks for people with this condition.

The co-dependent's need to please others makes it difficult to say "No" to risky sexual or drug-related behaviors. Achieving behavior change may be nearly impossible if people make judgments based on what their partners choose rather than on their own choices. Commitments to abide by safer sex guidelines are easily challenged when a co-dependent's partner threatens to leave rather than use a condom or latex barrier.

Many alcoholics struggle with issues of co-dependency. While this may not be the primary focus of their recovery, it is a matter that must be addressed when exploring HIV prevention.

Follow-Up Information

I have other questions you haven't discussed here. Where can I get answers?

There are telephone hotlines for questions about HIV disease. The numbers for the National AIDS Hotline are: 800-342-AIDS and 800-344-SIDA (information in Spanish).

There are also a number of local HIV-related information services. The National AIDS Hotline may be able to identify local resources for further information.

References

1. Stone KM, Peterson HB. Spermicides, HIV, and the vaginal sponge. *Journal of the American Medical Association.* 1992; 268(4): 521-523.
2. Gershon RRM, Vlahov D, Nelson KE. The risk of transmission of HIV-1 through non-percutaneous, non-sexual modes—a review. *AIDS.* 1990; 4(7): 645-650.
3. Lemp GF, Hirozawa AM, Cohen JB, et al. Survival for women and men with AIDS. *Journal of Infectious Diseases.* 1992; 166(July): 74-79.
4. Martin NL, Levy JA, Legg H, et al. Detection of infection with human immunodeficiency virus (HIV) type 1 in infants by an anti-HIV immunoglobulin A assay using recombinant proteins. *Journal of Pediatrics.* 1991; 118(3): 354-358.
5. Kaslow RA, Blackwelder WC, Ostrow DG, et al. No evidence for a role of alcohol or other psychoactive drugs in accelerating immunodeficiency in HIV-1 positive individuals. *Journal of the American Medical Association.* 1989; 261(23): 3424-3429.

CHAPTER FIVE

TALKING ABOUT SEXUALITY

IN THIS CHAPTER:

- The Importance of Talking about Sexuality
- Changes in Sexuality during Early Sobriety
- Counseling about Sexuality
- Beginning to Talk
- What to Talk about
- Slippery Spots for Providers: The Thirteenth Step
- What's Next?

CHAPTER FIVE

SEXUALITY

The Importance of Talking about Sexuality

In my own early recovery, my counselors encouraged me to "celebrate" my sexuality, but I didn't know how to do that. They supported me being out as a lesbian, but I couldn't talk openly about the women and men I'd had sex with in my life, or what I had done sexually. I was afraid of being judged. I avoided the particulars of my sexual life, even when this had some direct bearing on my recovery and sobriety. And no one really helped me understand how I could talk about sex in relation to recovery. It was years before I had a sense of how to do this.

Now I'm a recovery counselor myself. I remember these experiences when I talk about sex and HIV disease with participants. I know the way I went through this process isn't a good way today. We can't give participants the luxury of time to break through their denial about HIV-related risk or to get around to dealing with sexual issues. We've got to help people in early recovery figure this stuff out, and do it quickly.

It's more complicated than it used to be. But we're only living in our own denial if we don't move now to deal with HIV education and sexuality in early recovery.

– Recovery Counselor, Outpatient Clinic

If participants are going to learn about HIV prevention, providers are going to have to talk to them about sexuality. It's that simple.

But, talking about sexuality with people in recovery is not necessarily easy, and it can bring up conflicts for providers. They may find, for example, that discussing sexual practices with clients or participants contradicts professional training or philosophy. They may believe that they lack adequate knowledge about sexuality to be able to discuss it. And some providers may fear that discussions about sex, especially during early recovery, give mixed messages to participants who should be focusing on sobriety, not on sexuality.

The HIV epidemic has changed the ways in which providers must approach sexuality with alcoholics in recovery. It is critical that people in early recovery be clearly informed about HIV-related risks and understand their own sexual identity. Without this knowledge and understanding, there is little chance they will successfully follow safer sex guidelines. The difficulties of this change for providers are outweighed by the urgent need to help people cope with sexuality in the age of AIDS.

Changes in Sexuality during Early Sobriety

Many alcoholics in early recovery have never had sex without using alcohol or other substances. Sexual experiences are inextricably linked with their history and experience of drinking. It may be difficult for some to even think of sex as something that can happen in sobriety.

When an alcoholic becomes sober, chances are overwhelming that he or she will experience some change in sexual practice and functioning. Changes associated with drinking affect both the physical and emotional aspects of sexual experience. These effects often persist for some time in sobriety—from a few months to several years. Men often experience difficulty reaching orgasm, or achieving or maintaining erections. They may also have decreased sexual desire. Changes in hormonal balance caused by drinking may lead to gynecomastia (enlargement of the breasts), the loss of body hair and muscle tone, and the decrease in size of the testicles.

Women in early sobriety have reported decreased sexual desire, vaginismus—vaginal spasm—diminished vaginal lubrication, and painful intercourse. For both men and women, impaired spinal reflexes can interfere with sexual sensation and nerve function. The individual may be unable to register soft or gentle touch, or may actually feel physical discomfort during touching or other close contact.

The newly sober individual may experience great fatigue or anxiety, anemia, peripheral neuropathy—pain in the arms and legs—and other physical symptoms or illnesses. It is difficult, and in many cases impossible, for people with such conditions to have positive sexual experiences.

There are individuals in early sobriety who, for the first time, have strong sexual feelings and attractions. These feelings can be confusing or frightening, or they may be delightful and pleasant. They may also be distracting, and participants may feel frustrated at what they perceive to be limited options for gratifying sexual desires.

The sexual process can resonate with more general feelings common in sobriety. Participants experiencing low self-esteem and feelings of inadequacy may find these states intensified when faced with their own limited knowledge of normal sexual behavior or function, or confusion about their own sexual responses. Shame, guilt, and regret over past behaviors often extend to sexuality as well as alcohol use, and control issues may be heightened for participants who fear losing control while having sexual thoughts and experiences.

Because alcoholics tend to experience slowed emotional development while they are drinking, sexual feelings in sobriety bring up a range of immature responses. A 35-year-old man may find himself acting like a 12-year-old boy as he becomes aware of sexual attractions, thinks about asking someone out on a date, or suffers rejection by someone who does not return his affections.

Sex in sobriety can be a matter of considerable pain, embarrassment, and suffering. Fortunately, with information, patience, and support, recovery participants can also find a path to healing and self-love through a greater understanding of their sexual issues.

Counseling about Sexuality

Talking about sexuality can be difficult for both provider and participant. There is a special vulnerability each experiences during discussions of such personal matters. The work, however, is likely to be easier and more effective if some general principles are kept in mind.

Each of us is a sexual being, and sexuality can be a positive aspect of self-identity and recovery. Many alcoholics have engaged in self-destructive behaviors involving sexuality, and many have been victimized sexually by family members, friends, and strangers. They may have hurt others in sexual activities. The process of recovery often includes waves of memories or realizations about past sexual experiences that can be very painful.

These realizations bring individuals face to face with the breadth of their sexual experience and identity—for example, as victims, survivors, or perpetrators of abuse; as men or women; as gay, heterosexual, or bisexual people; and as individuals capable of enjoying sexual pleasures and afraid of the emotions that accompany sex. For some people, it seems easier to deny or avoid sexual identity, rather than to come to terms with these past experiences. Sex was something they did when they were drinking, it got them into trouble, and in sobriety they would just as soon avoid thinking about such situations.

Everyone is a sexual being, however, and sexual identity is an important part of who a person is. This does not mean that people must be sexually active, but it does mean that they can understand their behavior and who they are in a larger sense by understanding how they express their sexuality. Accepting the sexual self is also an essential step in building self-esteem and self-acceptance.

Discussions of sexuality can help people in recovery develop healthier ways of thinking about sex and acting on sexual feelings. Most alcoholics in early recovery, and many in later recovery, think about sex, or put energy into *not* thinking about sex. Avoidance of sexual issues, or denial that they exist, interferes with the development of rigorous honesty and thorough acceptance in recovery.

Providers can have discussions with participants about sex in sobriety, acknowledge and validate the issues likely to arise for recovering alcoholics, and emphasize the need to act responsibly concerning sexual behaviors. In such interactions, providers have an opportunity to help participants learn more about appropriate social and sexual behaviors. For example, it will be a new experience for many to have sexual feelings, to acknowledge such feelings, and to choose consciously neither to act on them, nor to drink as a way to blunt them.

DISCUSSIONS OF SEXUALITY AND SAFER SEX REINFORCE HONESTY AND SAVE LIVES. Some providers may feel that discussing sexuality is, in itself, opening a door to difficult emotions for the newly sober. Some programs reinforce this attitude and discourage discussions of sexual topics. But, people in recovery need support learning to talk honestly and directly about their own experiences and concerns. Discussions about sex make it more possible for the alcoholic in sobriety to follow guidelines that will protect him or her from HIV infection.

Many lives have already been saved by reviewing HIV information in the context of discussions about sexuality. By offering participants the opportunity to understand their own sexuality and to save their own lives, providers demonstrate respect and caring for them.

DISCUSSIONS OF SEXUALITY AND SAFER SEX SHOULD BE PAIRED WITH CLEAR MESSAGES ABOUT PROTECTING SOBRIETY AND FOCUSING ON RECOVERY. Alcoholism is a life-threatening disease. Maintaining sobriety saves lives. Sobriety is an essential focus in any program of recovery.

When providers encourage alcoholics in recovery to explore their own sexual issues and learn more about sex and safer sex, they must also emphasize the need to avoid situations that might lead to drinking. Most recovery providers would recommend, for example, that individuals in early sobriety make no major life changes if possible. Providers often believe it is best to avoid new sexual relationships during the first year of sobriety in order to "keep the focus on your recovery."

While this is a good idea, many do not heed this advice. Open and informative discussions of sex and sobriety may actually help participants stay more focused on their sobriety because they are given an opportunity to understand, validate, and process their own sexual issues. Behavioral guidelines recommending sexual abstinence in early recovery make more sense when offered as part of an open discussion about sexuality.

PROVIDERS ARE MOST EFFECTIVE WHEN THEY ARE NON-JUDGMENTAL ABOUT SEXUAL PREFERENCES AND PRACTICES. It is important for providers to accept people in recovery as they are. By modeling such acceptance, providers can help recovering alcoholics learn more about accepting and loving themselves. At the same time, providers also want to give honest feedback to participants, and may sometimes feel a need to confront an alcoholic on behaviors or attitudes that threaten sobriety.

Providers must think carefully about when to practice acceptance and when to confront a participant about issues related to sexuality. Sometimes, personal judgments guide a provider's behavior and interfere with efforts to support sobriety. In terms of sexual practices, providers may have judgments about such issues as homosexuality or bisexuality; having more than one sexual partner; going to sex clubs or to socials to have sex; having sex for pleasure, without love or emotional attachment; using vibrators, dildoes or other sex toys; and having sex with casual acquaintances.

Nothing about these practices themselves conflicts with sobriety or a commitment to recovery. The alcoholic's attitudes and feelings about the activity are more pertinent than the provider's. When working with participants on sexual issues, evaluate such situations carefully, help build positive feelings about sexuality, maintain the participant's trust by avoiding judgmental comments, and keep the focus on recovery.

Beginning to Talk

Discussions about sexuality are difficult for most people, not just for providers working with people in recovery. The greatest key to success is to make a sincere effort and to keep trying. With practice and experience, it becomes easier.

Sexuality can be discussed in an appropriate and constructive manner in many different settings. It might be easiest to arrange such discussions in groups. For example, sexuality or HIV prevention can be a topic of discussion at recovery home support groups; outpatient counseling groups; or 12-step meetings or conferences. Outside speakers who are knowledgeable about sex and sobriety or HIV transmission and safer sex might make a presentation to a support group or conference. An ongoing workshop on health issues might focus in some sessions on issues of sexual health and HIV prevention. (See also Appendix D: *Participant Training Tools* for a training on safer sex and HIV prevention.)

It may also be useful to discuss sexuality in individual sessions, such as psychotherapy or counseling. In this setting, however, the work is sometimes more complicated. Providers practicing conventional psychotherapy may feel it is inappropriate to initiate discussions of sexual practice or behavior. Participants may exhibit discomfort if counselors bring up the topic.

Many people in recovery have never been able to talk openly about sexuality with a person who did not intend to exploit them sexually. The opportunity to have a private discussion about sex with a trusted advisor can be new and confusing. Participants may respond with anger, fear, or romantic or sexual feelings. In these situations, participants may demonstrate a wide range of behaviors, including withdrawal, hostility, acting out, regression, or flirtatious behavior towards providers.

Despite these potential problems, however, it is useful for providers to learn to facilitate discussions of sexual issues with participants. In both individual and group settings, such discussions can offer participants an opportunity to learn socially appropriate responses to sexual feelings, to improve their skills talking about sexuality, and to expand their acceptance of the range of sexual expression. This can lead to a greater sense of empowerment and self-determination, and it is likely that such individuals will be more capable of making healthy sexual decisions.

Providers will want to build trust with participants with whom discussions of sexuality are taking place. It will always be essential for providers to maintain scrupulous boundaries. This includes respecting confidentiality, withholding judgment, and avoiding ridicule of participants' concerns or experiences.

Providers need to assess their own familiarity with these issues, as well as new or improved skills they may need to deal with these challenges. For example, how does a counselor respond if a participant expresses a sexual or romantic attraction to the counselor, another provider, or another participant?

There is a wide range of circumstances under which such feelings may occur and be expressed. No single approach will be appropriate in all of these situations. In general, providers will want to acknowledge and validate the feelings of participants, while gently clarifying the distinctions between having feelings and acting on them. Such participants are likely to need help understanding why acting on these feelings will not serve the process of recovery.

Within an inpatient, outpatient, or residential program, acting on attractions towards other participants will also interfere with the recovery focus. Two examples make this clear. First, progress in recovery is greater when defined roles and boundaries exist between providers and participants. Once romantic or sexual feelings are acted upon, these boundaries become blurred.

Second, sexual feelings often arise for participants in concert with many types of emotion. It is not unusual for participants in early recovery to sexualize their feelings of gratitude toward providers: their responses to caring and concern may be limited to emotions more akin to those associated with sexual attraction. When providers comment on this process, set appropriate limits, and demonstrate other ways of caring, participants are able to expand the range of their possible responses. Helping participants to identify their feelings and old patterns, and to establish new and healthy ones is an essential part of building sobriety.

Such interchanges between counselors and participants are delicate and require great sensitivity on the part of providers. The feelings of participants are often powerful and do not subside quickly or easily, and the intervention process may unfold over a period of days or weeks. Providers can gain further understanding and guidance in these circumstances by talking about their experiences with colleagues or mentors, reading on the topic, or attending relevant workshops at conferences.

What to Talk about

I was invited to come into a program of early recovery, as a consultant, and provide a support and educational group about HIV risk, safer sex, and related issues. I'm a person in recovery myself, I've worked in recovery settings, and I'm a staff member of an AIDS agency now, so I felt well-prepared for the group. But issues came up that I had not anticipated.

There were a lot of questions I had to answer before I even got started. Who was going to participate in the group? Was each person ready to address the material we would cover? Did staff understand the nature of this group and the intense responses participants might have? Was there someone at the agency who was able to co-facilitate the group with me and was trusted by the residents? Was the agency really ready to address these issues, or were unresolved internal problems going to set the project up for failure?

Some people think doing AIDS education, and supporting people in changing their behaviors, means covering the basic facts about HIV transmission and prevention, and that's it. I don't believe this. People need to explore their own histories, understandings, and motivations to develop the tools necessary to change these very personal behaviors. This can involve some pretty intense interactions within a group.

Once I was actually doing the group, it was particularly challenging to find the fine line between dealing appropriately and honestly with the realities of HIV disease and catapulting participants into slippery places at a time when their coping skills were very limited. When talking about AIDS, we talked about life-threatening illness, grief, loss, the nitty gritty about sex, needle use—very hard issues in the best of circumstances.

I think the group was successful, and the people who participated said it was helpful. But I learned something else about this process: if you have something in mind for the group, and then it doesn't feel like the right time for that idea, just change it. To use a program cliché, "Easy does it (when reviewing your expectations), but do it!"

– AIDS Counselor

Sexual topics span a spectrum from concrete and specific issues to deeper, personal concerns. In this section, several categories of topics are described to help providers prepare for this process. In real life, however, the work will not fall into such neat divisions.

Concrete Issues

Many people in recovery have little education about the mechanics of sexuality. To begin, providers can help them understand basic sexual anatomy. What are the male and female sexual parts? What is the human sexual response cycle, and what role does each anatomical part play in sexual response? Clarify that everyone has his or her own range of sexual response, which may look similar to or different from that of others.

Sexual health is a new concept for many alcoholics in recovery. Participants can be educated about the need for regular gynecologic check-ups for women, breast and testicular self-exams, the use of condoms or other latex barriers to avoid exposure to sexually transmitted diseases (including HIV), and how to seek medical care for sexual health problems. Some of this information might have to be communicated in basic terms. For example, telling someone, "Condom use is important!" will not be as effective as taking time to explain how condoms are properly used, and giving participants an opportunity to talk about and practice condom use in a non-sexual setting. (See also Appendix D: *Participant Training Tools* for information about condom and latex barrier education.)

Deeper Personal Issues

Typically, discussions of "concrete" sexual matters, such as safer sex or the sexual response cycle, will bring up personal feelings and recollections of past experiences. These can be complex or confusing, and participants may feel uncomfortable or awkward, especially if they believe they are poorly informed on the topic, or if they feel different from others in their social or support network. Straightforward discussions of sexual activities may stimulate feelings of guilt about past behaviors or conflicts about current desires.

Participants can find themselves in challenging places in terms of sobriety or safer sex as these thoughts or feelings occur to them. Providers who are attentive to these processes can help participants progress in their recovery.

A review of HIV-related risk activities, for example, might bring a participant to the sudden realization that he has had some HIV-related risk in the past. He may feel guilt or shame about his past behaviors, anger at himself or others, or fear. Along with this realization comes anxiety about his current antibody status—does he have HIV infection? How this person handles his anxiety will probably reflect his current progress in recovery. Does he have tools he can use to help him cope? Are others in his recovery community able to support him as he works through these issues? Is his program strong enough to keep him focused on his recovery?

It is natural that participants experience a range of deeper feelings in response to sex education sessions. In group settings, one participant's sharing of such feelings may open the way for a more meaningful discussion for the whole group. In a group reviewing safer sex guidelines, for example, one member may begin to discuss the question of sexual motivation—why he or she has sex in the first place. Soon others may explore their own motivations for having sex, and this full group discussion can help members develop greater insight into their own and others' behaviors.

Providers can also facilitate this deeper level of discussion by focusing on a topic likely to be of concern to an individual or group. For example, discussions of sexuality can lead to an examination of personal boundaries. Is it possible for people to maintain strong personal boundaries in sexually intimate relationships? Is it necessary or desirable to do so? Can they say "no" to partners who want to engage in unsafe sex?

Matters of personal choice and self-esteem can also serve as a useful focus. How can participants develop the skills necessary to make their own choices about their sexual lives and relationships? Is some minimum level of self-esteem necessary before a person can insist on safer sex with a partner who would prefer not to follow those guidelines?

Among people who have lost friends to HIV disease, discussions of sexuality also bring up issues of grief and loss. Sex is linked, symbolically and in reality, to illness and death. Providers can help participants articulate or identify this experience of grief and express some of the sadness they feel.

Participants may "act out" during discussions of sexuality, making crude comments, sexist or racist remarks, or sexual innuendoes. All of these actions provide material for deeper discussion of the issues, as well as an opportunity to model and support socially appropriate behavior.

Recovery issues

Discussions of sexuality offer a considerable opportunity to explore larger recovery issues and help participants anticipate and respond to potential problems. Many tools useful in other areas of recovery can be applied to sexual matters as well, and providers can help participants understand how to use these tools.

For example, a helpful slogan for the recovering alcoholic feeling an impulse to drink is, "Think through the drink." The slogan encourages the individual to stop and think about what it would be like to take the drink, what he or she might do after the first drink, how this would feel, what would happen next, and so on. Taking the time to stop and think can help someone realize that acting on the impulse would be a destructive step, a step backward in recovery.

A similar process can be applied to sexual feelings or impulses. What would it be like to act on the impulse? What would happen afterwards? How would the person feel? Such questions help a participant clarify the choices a situation offers, and what course of action would be best.

Other recovery tools can also be adapted for sexual issues. A participant might want to work on a personal inventory of his or her sexual history, following the guidelines offered in AA literature for completing the Fourth Step* but keeping the focus on sexual history, behavior, and attitudes. Or, a participant might find it helpful to think about the step on which he or she is currently working and what that step suggests about sexual issues or concerns.

Flooding of Memories

Some participants may run headlong into sexual concerns in the first few days of sobriety; others may find that sexual issues arise with a sudden and fierce insistence only after five years of recovery.

---

* The Fourth Step of Alcoholics Anonymous: "Made a searching and fearless moral inventory of ourselves."

Providers can expect such matters to come up at varying points in the recovery process, although they tend to be especially powerful in the first year of sobriety.

Most striking in this light is the flooding of memories that occurs as individuals stop using alcohol or other drugs to mask feelings or experiences. They may remember incest or sexual abuse, rape, or other forms of sexual violence, and may have been either victims or perpetrators, or both. Old experiences that seemed resolved suddenly arise again bringing new memories of terrible pain or fear. Details of past experiences emerge with greater detail, accuracy, and intrusiveness.

Such powerful feelings, especially if they are unfamiliar, present a challenge to people in recovery. Strong emotions demand attention and may seem uncontrollable. Under these conditions, the situation can feel all consuming, and participants may fear loss of control of self and surroundings. Drinking had provided the illusion over the years that feelings were under control, and drinking may again become appealing in such situations. Great and unfamiliar pain brings into question the whole process of recovery. "If it's going to hurt this much, why bother?" Participants may experience all of this turmoil at an unconscious level, but providers must be alert to the possibility that participants may relapse under these circumstances.

There is controversy about when during an individual's recovery such powerful issues should be addressed, and there is no clear answer to this question. It could be reasonably argued that addressing an incest history at six months sobriety may increase the likelihood of relapse. By the same token, however, it could be argued that *not* addressing such an issue increases relapse potential. These matters must be evaluated on a case-by-case basis, and participants should take an active role in deciding the course of the work.

It is helpful to collaborate with participants in identifying these deeper issues and encourage them to develop some kind of "container" for their experiences. This might simply mean that provider and participant acknowledge that an event happened, and that the participant has been able to share the memory, even in a limited way, with another person. Some participants will benefit from writing out a Fourth Step on the experience. For others, in-depth work on an issue can be set aside while participants focus on building strength in their recovery program.

Identity Issues

Success in recovery will be based, in part, on the development of a complete sense of self—the perception of oneself as a whole person, with feelings, faults, and virtues. It involves accepting oneself as an imperfect, but improving, person. Participants will not be able to develop this perception if they are avoiding key components of self identity.

Some matters related to personal sexuality touch on core issues of identity. Core identity can be described as any aspect of personal identity so essential to a person's self perception that he or she is incomplete without it. In sobriety, alcoholics who have denied or neglected matters of core identity in the past often find themselves re-examining, in a very profound sense, who they are and what life means to them.

Precisely what constitutes a core issue varies from person to person. Imagine, for example, two men sitting together in a room. Both are alcoholics in recovery, both are Catholic, both are fathers. One of them describes his Catholicism as a casual family practice that never affected him deeply. He no longer attends Mass and has no particular religious interest. His Catholicism has little to do with his sense of self, of who he is.

The other man speaks with tremendous bitterness and anger about the pain and degradation he experienced growing up Catholic. Even today, he struggles with a sense of shame about himself, which he ascribes to his Catholic upbringing. In sobriety, he finds himself often thinking about his sinfulness, and he cannot imagine how to escape these terrible thoughts without drinking. His Catholicism has a great deal to do with his sense of identity, and his inability to resolve the conflicts he feels may jeopardize his recovery.

The first man, speaking of fatherhood, is delighted by his daughter, deeply concerned for her, and states that his entire sense of what was important to the world, and to him as an individual, changed the day she was born. Part of what brings him to recovery is his wish to have a healthy relationship with her. He could never separate his identity as a father from his sense of who he is.

The second fathered two children as a teenager, has not seen the children or their mother for the past 10 years, and rarely thinks about any of them. Being a father is an incidental part of his personal history and not directly related to his core identity at this time.

In the realm of sexual identity and experience, sexual orientation will often represent a core issue, especially for lesbians, gay men, or bisexuals. If participants cannot come to terms with being gay or bisexual, the strength of their recovery will be compromised. Many who do well in the first months of recovery later relapse as unresolved issues of sexual orientation intrude more and more into their lives. These situations are especially difficult for gay and bisexual people experiencing homophobia in their programs or recovery communities.

Discussions of sexuality may touch on other core issues. For one person, it might involve being a survivor of incest or sexual abuse. For women, considerations of power and submission often arise—sexual experience may be a metaphor for broader relationship styles. A person with HIV disease who thinks about accepting him or herself sexually also has an opportunity to practice more general self-acceptance.

Participants and providers alike will want to be aware of the ways in which the decision to address, or not address, a core issue of identity affects sobriety and recovery. As with the flooding of memories mentioned above, it is especially important to consider whether moving too quickly in exploring a core issue, or avoiding the matter altogether, contributes to the likelihood of relapse.

As discussions of HIV disease and sexuality become more common in recovery settings, so will participants' struggles with these kinds of issues. With consistency and support from providers, participants can clarify and consolidate self image, integrate personal identities, and develop greater acceptance of themselves. The practical application of 12-step principles to discussions of sexual concerns has the potential to help people facing such complex issues move forward in their recovery, each in his or her own time.

Slippery Spots for Providers: the Thirteenth Step

People who practice AA's Twelve Steps often joke about the "Thirteenth Step": using familiarity with the Twelve Steps to attract a person who is less knowledgeable about the program into a sexual or romantic relationship. This kind of activity is not at all consistent with the principles of AA. Mention of the Thirteenth Step draws attention to the problems that can arise when a more experienced individual lets a sexual attraction divert him or her from personal and program goals.

Thirteenth Step tendencies can easily arise, even in the work of conscientious providers. Participants who are learning about their sexual selves, who are coming to terms with past experiences of sexual pain, who are beginning to rejoice in the freedom recovery offers, often touch providers deeply. At such moments, interactions with participants can be open and loving, and leave them feeling vulnerable. It is not surprising, then, that providers sometimes feel attraction to participants. This is a natural occurrence, especially when discussions of sexual matters are taking place.

It is also natural that participants sometimes develop romantic or sexual feelings towards those who have helped them in their recovery, who have listened to them carefully, who understand their experiences. Such attractions may become more evident in a setting where sexuality is discussed forthrightly.

These natural attractions, however, can lead providers to difficulties. Providers need to keep their own motives, issues, and roles very clear. The boundaries between provider and participant provide an essential component of the healing and recovery process. In situations where these boundaries become indistinct, that process is in danger of being compromised.

Of course, providers should not develop romantic or sexual relationships with participants with whom they work. But providers must also give special attention to more subtle interactions with participants that could be experienced as flirtatious or seductive. For example, participants should not be teased about sexual or romantic matters, and the confidentiality of sexual information shared must be respected.

Recovery providers are encouraged to discuss these issues with colleagues in an ongoing way. If romantic or sexual attraction towards a participant seems to be developing, speak sincerely with a trusted consultant or advisor. It is not necessary to be hard on oneself for having warm feelings for participants or clients. It is, however, essential to be rigorous in examining the nature of behaviors with participants and maintaining appropriate boundaries.

What's Next?

The HIV epidemic and the need to discuss sexual matters, even in early recovery, place new demands on recovery providers. Most providers naturally resist adding more complicated obligations to their work; there was already more than enough to do before this epidemic developed.

Recovery participants have always presented complex concerns to providers. While HIV infection brings new and urgent demands to discussions of sexuality in recovery, the conflicts, confusion, and challenges that arise have been there all along. HIV disease deepens these, but it does not create them.

What the HIV epidemic does generate is an urgency about the need for participants, even early in recovery, to come to terms with sexual experience and personal sexual issues. Providers who can look at their own fears and apprehensions about this work, as well as limitations in knowledge and skills, can take action to improve their ability to counsel and educate about sexuality and HIV disease. Provider awareness and willingness are among the most important tools in helping participants learn to consider their own sexual issues. (See also Appendix D: *Participant Training Tools* for more information about HIV transmission and safer sex education.) Ultimately, these will also be some of the essential elements that contribute to the slowing, and with hope, the ending of this epidemic.

CHAPTER SIX

CULTURE AND ATTITUDE

In This Chapter:

- Culture and Cultural Norms
- Exploring "Cultural Thresholds"
- Culture and HIV Counseling
- Attitude
- Relapse
- Responding to Negative Attitudes
- On Reflection: Culture and Attitude

CHAPTER SIX

CULTURE AND ATTITUDE

Everyone has his or her own way of talking about the sensitive and difficult topics that arise when dealing with HIV disease. People learn about these topics and how to discuss them, partly through their cultures—the groups with whom they have lived and from whom they have developed identity. When people discuss emotional topics—sexuality, drug use, illness, and death—with people from cultures different from their own, they may be especially likely to misunderstand, to offend, or to be ineffective in their efforts to communicate.

A person's approach to sensitive issues is also determined partly by attitude—beliefs formed from personal experience and learning. Attitudes may contribute to or interfere with an understanding of other people and with the ability to communicate.

Culture and Cultural Norms

My girlfriend, who is Latina, accompanied me on a visit to my Anglo family. My mom was preparing dinner, I was fixing a salad, and my girlfriend was just sitting there reading the newspaper. When it was time to set the table, I asked her to help out. She seemed indignant and, although she did help, she was not very gracious about it.

When I talked to her later, I told her I was angry that she had been so uncooperative about setting the table. My mom and I had been rushing around like crazy to get dinner ready, and in my family everyone always pitches in with the last-minute preparations.

She said she was angry, too. In her family, a guest was always treated with great respect. They would never have asked a visitor to help prepare the table or clean up after dinner. She considered my request discourteous and disrespectful.

So without even knowing it or really meaning it, both of us had felt that we had been slighted and hurt.

– AIDS Educator

In HIV-related work, a broad definition of culture is useful.* In this context, culture is not the same thing as ethnicity or race. While ethnicity and race are important influences, gender, class, educational experience, sexual orientation, political affiliation, and career are among the factors that also affect culture. At its most basic, culture is a group's "design for living"—the common assumptions about what is and what is not important, what are the goals and meaning of life, what is right and what is wrong, and how one should behave and how one expects others to behave.

When people from different cultures meet, they evaluate one another. They look, listen, smell, and taste the differences in their cultures. Then, they make the judgment: "Is this person like me or not like me?" The ability to trust a person who is culturally different depends on the perception of some commonality or on the acceptance of differences. For example, for a participant to trust a counselor perceived to be culturally different, the participant must identify some shared characteristic with the counselor or sense an acceptance from the counselor of the differences between them.

The values learned from culture are often so deeply ingrained that people are not even aware of them. It is difficult to see the ways in which these values affect personal behavior especially in interactions among people whose cultural values are different. But in providing HIV-related education or counseling, awareness of cultural beliefs is an essential tool for success.

When providers are aware of their own values and judgments, they are better able to suspend them, if necessary, while working with someone whose culture and values are different. This does not mean providers should abandon personal beliefs or values. By setting them aside for a short while, however, providers may be able

---

* Many of the ideas presented in this section were originally formulated by Noel Day, Polaris Research and Development, San Francisco.

to communicate more effectively with participants. Some circumstances where this insight might be useful include:

- A provider is discussing the importance of using condoms for HIV prevention. A participant says that she is a Catholic and that using condoms would be a sin.
- A gay male participant is talking to a woman counselor about HIV disease. She is heterosexual, married, and her only sexual partner in her life has been her husband. The participant asks for detailed information about how to have sex safely with many anonymous partners.
- A lesbian counselor is talking to a self-identified lesbian participant. The participant says she is concerned about her HIV-related risk because she has recently had unprotected intercourse with a gay male friend. The counselor firmly believes that a woman who chooses to have sex with a man is not a lesbian and should not call herself a lesbian.
- A recovery counselor is working with an alcoholic in early recovery, discussing HIV-related risks. The alcoholic describes a long involvement with drug use, including injection drug use. The counselor believes his own expertise is in the field of alcoholism, and he does not like to work with people who have extensive drug histories.

In such situations, if a provider's own judgments are communicated, a participant's trust and willingness to share his or her thoughts may be compromised.

Exploring "Cultural Thresholds"

Providers might think of some of these instances as "cultural thresholds"—places rich in variety and sensitivity where different cultures meet. To reach people who have backgrounds different from our own, to communicate effectively, we must be able to cross these thresholds. Most people can cross certain thresholds easily, while other thresholds can only be crossed with great effort. What is easy and what is difficult will vary from person to person.

Take a moment to think about some of your own cultural norms right now. Which thresholds are easy for you to cross, and which are more challenging? You can take a simple inventory for yourself by reading slowly down the list below and thinking about how comfortable you are when faced by a person who differs from you in the following ways:

- Sexual orientation
- Class
- Political beliefs
- Religious or spiritual beliefs
- Educational background
- Ethnic background
- Race
- Gender
- Age
- Beliefs about recovery

As you reflect on these areas, also think about whether it is easier for you to cross the threshold in one direction than in another. For example, a middle class woman who identifies class as a threshold that is difficult might find it easier to cross that threshold with a person who is upper class than with someone who is poor or working class.

Because people are complex beings with many different qualities, some combinations of thresholds make the crossing easier or more difficult. The same middle class woman described above might find it easier to cross towards a working class woman than towards a working class man. In such an instance, the cultural influence of gender would clearly be important to her.

Culture and HIV Counseling

In talking about HIV education and counseling, many sensitive topics are raised. Perhaps the most immediate is sex. When providers assess HIV-related risk during a counseling session, they are asking participants to reveal intimate personal history. How does a provider respond if a participant uses unfamiliar terms or words the provider finds offensive? What expression does the participant see on the provider's face when describing sexual behaviors that are repugnant or strange to the provider? How patient can the provider be with someone who does not have words to describe his or her sexual practices? What phrases does the provider use to explain safer sex practices; are these terms the participant understands? How well can the provider cross this threshold with someone whose values or experience is different from his or her own?

People learning about HIV infection are also asked to think about issues of health, illness, and death. These, too, are emotionally charged areas, deeply affected by cultural differences. The importance of seeking medical care; the proper way to treat people who are ill; who bears the responsibility when an individual becomes ill; what is the best course of medical treatment for an illness—people will respond differently to each of these topics.

A provider schooled in Western medicine will probably take for granted the cause-and-effect relationship of HIV-related risk behaviors and HIV transmission. If a person has unsafe sex with someone who has HIV disease, he or she is obviously at risk for HIV infection. However, this belief may not make much sense to someone who has other ideas about the causality of illness. Perhaps illness is seen as a punishment from God, a matter of inevitable fate, or a consequence of past generations' misdeeds. If providers can perceive the backdrop of their own cultural norms—which they may take for granted—they may be able to detach from those beliefs and recognize a different point of view. When this occurs, it becomes possible for providers to have productive discussions with participants whose world views are quite different.

Providers are encouraged to think carefully about norms and differences, and to learn more about their own cultural norms. Staff groups can review the list of "thresholds" above, completing a staff inventory similar to the "group inventory" practiced in some 12-step meetings. An outside facilitator familiar with cultural issues in HIV-related and recovery work might help in this process. Differences in values, language, and belief are inevitable when good HIV education is offered. It is essential that providers keep these differences in mind and do their best to bridge the gaps that arise. (See also Appendix E: *Provider Training Tools* for a staff inservice on "Exploring and Understanding Cultural Norms.")

Attitude

An alcoholic I'd known ages ago came to me to do a Ninth Step. He said he felt he owed me an amends. This was news to me! He was always someone I'd felt good about—definitely okay. I was glad to see he was still sober and working a recovery program.*

"My amends," he told me, "is about what I didn't say back at the house. We always joked around and talked like we were it: different, better than the others. Like, 'We're all the same, but not really.' I was as guilty as the next guy—telling stories about 'fruits' in my shares and all...

"Well, I'm ashamed that I did that. When I told those stories, played along, I felt like I couldn't be sure that something I shared myself—about someone I cared about, anything really personal—might not some day be turned into those jokes and stories. I wasn't honest, not the way I really needed to be."

So this guy's amends was about not being honest, and I got it. I really did. My attitude stank back then, and this guy was living proof of it. He couldn't come clean with things because he was worried I'd judge him. And that affected his sobriety.

I know I'm not responsible if another guy drinks, but this made me think. I hope I don't do something like that again. I'm trying not to. And, if I see other people I work with or know doing the same thing, I let them know about my experience.

– Former Counselor, Alcohol Recovery Home

Like culture, attitude—belief formed from experience and learning—influences the success of HIV education and counseling. For this reason, providers should strive to be aware of any of their own attitudes that might interfere with efforts to educate or counsel participants about HIV disease. Attitudes that frequently arise when addressing alcoholism, such as denial, control, or blame, also often

---

* The Ninth Step of Alcoholics Anonymous: "Made direct amends to such people whenever possible, except when to do so would injure them or others." "Such people" refers to "persons we had harmed," mentioned in the Eighth Step.

appear when discussing HIV-related issues. Not surprisingly, attitudes that have contributed to progress in recovery—acceptance, patience, and keeping things simple and focused—have also proven helpful in HIV work.

There is a tried and true process used by people in recovery to identify their own negative or destructive attitudes about drinking and alcoholism, even when these attitudes are unconscious. This involves the observation of behavior in a situation related to drinking or alcohol. For example, the wife of an alcoholic, repeatedly calls his workplace to report that he is ill, explaining that he has the flu, a cold, food poisoning, or a bad back, when he actually has a hangover. She believes that by covering for his lateness or absence, she is expressing her love for him. She tells herself that in time this "love" will lead him to change his drinking patterns. The wife's behavior reveals two common, and misconceived, attitudes that arise with the disease of alcoholism:

- that someone other than the drinker—in this case, his wife—can control the person's drinking;
- that denying the severity of someone's alcoholism can help the situation.

If someone simply told this wife directly that she was in denial about her husband's alcoholism and that her endeavor to control his behavior would be fruitless, she would probably disagree. If, however, someone was able to discuss her behavior with her in a careful, non-judgmental way, she would more likely see that she did have attitudes concerning control and denial that were actually enabling her husband's drinking. Naming the attitudes—the wife's control and denial responses—is less effective in changing the situation than displaying the attitudes in action by exploring her behavior.

In HIV-related work, behaviors provide a similar "window" through which attitudes can be observed. For example, an alcohol recovery provider refuses to read a handout on HIV disease. Asked about his behavior, he explains, "This information is not relevant to the work I do. HIV will not affect the kind of people I work with." His behavior and comments demonstrate common attitudes in the disease of alcoholism. First, there is denial: the HIV epidemic cannot affect alcoholics in recovery. Second, there is a mythology about what kind of people are affected by HIV disease, just as there are false beliefs about what kind of people are alcoholics. There is also an implied negative judgment about people who might get HIV.

As with the alcoholic's wife described above, however, if someone simply told this provider that he was demonstrating denial, false beliefs, and negative judgments, he might well disagree. If, on the other hand, he willingly engaged in a discussion and examination of his behavior, he might recognize on his own that some of these attitudes were both present and counterproductive.

Providers who are themselves in recovery will want to pay special attention to their attitudes about HIV disease, because these will often mirror the attitudes they experienced during periods of active using as well as in recovery. In the same way that these attitudes create obstacles on the path to recovery, they will interfere with the ability to work effectively and appropriately with HIV infection. Because providers are often particularly talented at screening out their own faulty thinking, negative attitudes about HIV disease are likely to intrude in a subtle way. Note behaviors, feelings, or thoughts that suggest the following:

- The HIV epidemic is not an issue for active alcoholics or those in recovery.
- We can control someone else's HIV-related risk behaviors.
- Other individuals are to blame for the HIV epidemic, and it is not an issue we need to be concerned with.
- Participants with HIV disease are to blame for their illness. They are bad people or have done something bad to become infected.
- People with HIV disease, or at known risk for HIV infection, are less important than other people. They will not benefit from a recovery program, and "we" have nothing in common with "them."
- Someone at risk for HIV infection must take the HIV antibody test; or someone with HIV disease must seek a particular kind of medical treatment. We know what is best for this person.

- We are special in some way. We, or the participants we work with, will be spared the dangers of the HIV epidemic even if we, or they, do not follow prevention guidelines.
- The situation is hopeless and there is nothing that we can do about it.

In the same way that some attitudes can alert providers to possible difficulties in offering sound HIV-related counseling and education, others can signal areas of strength and likely success. Providers will want to cultivate attitudes that reflect open-mindedness; acceptance of diverse beliefs, values, and lifestyles; willingness to acknowledge limitations as a provider (and to make appropriate referrals when necessary); and an understanding that both HIV infection and alcoholism are diseases, and that alcoholics and people with HIV disease deserve compassion, not blame.

Relapse

Alcoholism is a disease characterized by denial and relapse. Providers often use relapse as a learning tool for participants: a slip into drinking can offer an excellent illustration of alcoholism at work, and participants who do slip may be able to see this more clearly after they have spent some time in recovery.

Most recovery providers have found a balance that allows them to address relapse directly and clearly without being punitive. People with years of sobriety are fully willing to admit, "I am only one drink away from the alcoholic on the street."

Changing sexual behaviors to prevent the spread of HIV infection is a process also characterized by relapse. People who have changed behaviors to conform with safer sex guidelines may find it difficult to maintain these changes over time. As the epidemic continues, it is evident that relapse into unsafe sexual behaviors is a widespread phenomenon.

The recovery provider working with a participant who slips around sexual behaviors may face a particularly thorny challenge. Is this type of relapse different from a relapse around drinking? Should it be addressed in a similar or different manner? How does the provider feel about the participant who slips sexually, and what does the provider do in response? Does the provider feel differently if the participant is known to be HIV-infected?

Attitude will play an influential role in determining the response to questions like these. The Twelve Steps provide wisdom and experience that can be useful in thinking about sexual relapse. It is unlikely that a punitive or judgmental approach will support individuals in making new commitments to avoid unsafe sex. It will be more helpful to develop strategies that encourage participants to abide by those commitments one day at a time.

Responding to Negative Attitudes

I had an opportunity to work with a participant in my program who had been diagnosed with a life-threatening cancer pretty early in his recovery. This was a devastating experience for him. He was about my age, and his drinking history was similar to my own. I felt a lot of acceptance and understanding of his feelings. I would have felt the same fear, disappointment, and anger if this had happened to me right after I got sober.

I kept emphasizing the ways the tools of his program could help him live with his feelings, one day at a time. I shared some of the ideas that had really helped me early in my recovery. I felt very connected to him.

A few months after that, I was speaking to a participant in early recovery who had HIV disease. He was a gay man, and he had had many sexual partners in his life, he used to do poppers, and he shot speed a few times. All the while that I was talking to him, I kept thinking, "I have nothing in common with this man. I have no way of understanding what he is going through, or of helping him." I tried to be helpful, but I couldn't think of much to say.

I was really jolted later that evening when a co-worker I really trusted pointed out how differently I had behaved with these two men. Both of them were facing similar issues, and both of them needed support in their recovery. But my attitude about HIV disease and gay men made it impossible for me to share the same love and support with the second man that I had with the first. If I hadn't seen that difference in behavior, you would never have convinced me that

I had any prejudices or judgments about gay people or AIDS. And I wouldn't have been able to do anything to change the situation or improve my ability to help.

– Recovery Home Counselor

It is often stated in 12-step meetings, "If we do good things, good thoughts will follow." Alcoholics in recovery know well that "stinking thinking" leads to destructive behavior. It is especially true in early recovery that people must sidestep unhealthy thinking and do the footwork necessary to improve the course of recovery. Often this is done with the guidance of someone with longer term sobriety, and it is a skill that must continue to be used, one day at a time, for a lifetime.

These skills can be of immense value in HIV counseling as well. If, by examining behaviors, providers can identify negative or destructive thinking about participants with HIV-related concerns, they have the option of changing those behaviors. Where the behaviors change, a better attitude often follows. Providers can develop more positive attitudes about HIV disease by implementing the AA slogan "Awareness, Acceptance and Action."

Awareness. Providers can increase their awareness of HIV infection and its implications for the recovery community in a variety of ways: reading relevant books or articles, keeping up with news reports, and attending HIV-related workshops at conferences. Providers can heighten their awareness of their attitudes by carefully noticing how they behave in situations where HIV disease is a concern.

Acceptance. Acceptance of the importance and impact of HIV disease on the recovery community can be fostered by talking with HIV-infected people in recovery, and by listening to and validating participants' concerns about HIV disease. Acceptance of the existence of one's own mistaken attitudes can be improved by acknowledging imperfection in oneself, recognizing at the same time the capacity for self-improvement.

Action. Providers can take action to help in the HIV epidemic by working to educate participants and colleagues alike, by advocating for the interests of HIV-infected people in recovery, and by encouraging greater awareness of these issues in program settings and the recovery community at large. Action to improve negative attitudes about HIV disease can include acting "as if" we thought differently—choosing behaviors that reflect positive, supportive thinking about HIV-related issues.

On Reflection: Culture and Attitude

This chapter has suggested that providers endeavor to bridge, rather than alter, cultural differences. Attitudes, however, are subject to modification, especially by observing and evaluating behaviors. Can providers seek to influence values if these are based on cultural, rather than attitudinal, factors?

Culture is a phenomenon of groups. It is neither possible nor desirable to change or influence a cultural belief when working with individuals. The belief belongs to the culture, to a group of people, and cultures change only through group experience.

Attitude is an individual attribute, based on personal experience, often in tandem with cultural background. New experiences or learning can change attitude. Membership in new groups can give an individual exposure to different cultural values. As experience and cultures blend in individuals, each person develops his or her own unique characteristics and qualities.

It is at this individual level that explorations concerning cultural values and personal attitude can lead to change. The provider's role in this process is to determine whether change is essential to a participant's recovery.

Imagine, for example, a participant in a recovery program who habitually makes sexual remarks about women. Other participants, as well as counselors, dislike his sexist values. With the help of his counselors, this participant learns to modify his social behavior so he does not alienate other members of the program. However, consistent with the beliefs of the culture in which he was raised, he continues to feel that women are primarily useful as sexual objects. As objectionable as this may be to some providers, this belief does not interfere with this participant's ability to maintain his program of recovery. His providers have been successful in bridging this difference and supporting the participant in recovery.

In another example, a woman raised in an upper middle class community has been reared on values of community service and volunteerism. She has been taught that it is commendable to become involved in the problems of others, to lend support, and to help people get through their difficulties. When she enters recovery, she finds the troubles of other participants far more compelling than her own. She has an uncanny knack for offering people "pearls of wisdom" that help them make sense of their conflicts. Soon, participants are coming to her for support, often preferring her advice to that of their counselors or sponsors. She is very busy with this work. She helps others write out their Fourth Steps* but never gets around to writing her own.

The value of serving and helping others seems admirable, but this participant's progress is being hindered by her behaviors. This is an instance where exploration, and even confrontation, of attitude and belief is useful. It is not necessary for the participant to give up her values, but to succeed in her recovery efforts, she needs to change her attitudes and behaviors.

One of the wonderful things providers learn by participating in or observing the recovery process is that attitudes can change, and that changed attitudes can dramatically alter the quality of a person's life. By doing HIV-related work, providers can also see how their own changed attitudes can improve the efficacy and influence of their work. Attending to personal attitudes can help providers progress in their abilities to support participants and to have a meaningful impact on the HIV epidemic. At the same time, by respecting personal attitudes—and their foundations in culture and experience—providers can encourage useful change while enabling participants to maintain a stable world view during recovery, a time when so much else is in flux.

---

* The Fourth Step of Alcoholics Anonymous: "Made a searching and fearless moral inventory of ourselves."

CHAPTER SEVEN

LEGAL ISSUES FOR PROVIDERS

In This Chapter:

- Access to Services
- Confidentiality
- Duty to Warn and Permission to Warn
- Progressive Illness
- Harnessing the Law

CHAPTER SEVEN

LEGAL ISSUES FOR PROVIDERS

The HIV epidemic has presented service providers, including those serving people in recovery, with new laws that affect their practice. For their own protection, it is important for providers to be familiar with basic laws about non-discrimination, charting, confidentiality, and the duty to protect as they relate to HIV-related care.[1]

For many providers, the study of legal issues seems an unappealing task. The language and concepts are technical and often complex, and it may be difficult to see how a particular case or law relates to a provider's own situation. The idea that the HIV epidemic presents special laws that affect medical, mental health, and recovery settings can be especially discouraging.

It is useful to remember that the kinds of legal issues that have arisen concerning HIV disease are not, for the most part, new to recovery providers. The laws tend to address matters such as duty to protect (sometimes called "duty to warn"), confidentiality, infection control, access to services, and the presence of participants with progressive illnesses in a program. Legal issues, however, may arise more often with HIV-related participants, and areas of law that were ambiguous before may seem even more so when applied to HIV infection.

This chapter was written primarily by Gary James Wood, JD.

It does not present legal advice in regard to particular situations, but is meant solely as a guide to general situations in which the issues covered here may arise. For advice about specific circumstances, please consult a lawyer. The laws described in this chapter reflect the law as of April 1992. These laws are subject to substantial change through judicial interpretations, statutory amendment, and voter referendum.

There are a few important concepts related to HIV-related law that providers will want to note.

Unsettled and ambiguous law. Laws can and do change, and HIV-related laws, in particular, are currently unsettled. Ambiguous areas of HIV-related law are best explored by looking at laws in similar situations that are more settled, for example, other cases involving a progressive illness or the spread of a sexually transmitted disease.

Liability. In general, liability is determined, and may lead to legal penalties, when a deliberate or negligent action causes harm to another person. But liability is not necessarily determined in light of "right" and "wrong," nor does an absence of liability protect a provider from lawsuits. In the end, following the law may not keep you out of court, and acting irresponsibly may not mean you will be sued.

Variability. HIV-related laws vary from state to state. In some cases federal, rather than local, laws will regulate the behavior of an agency or an individual provider.

Ethics. Laws may conflict with a profession's or a provider's ethical standards. In these cases, providers or workplaces will have to make their own judgments about whether to adhere to the law or to what they believe is the right thing to do.

Access to Services

1. May a recovery program, or an individual provider, deny treatment to a person because he or she is known to have HIV disease?

- Providers shall not discriminate against HIV-infected people solely on the basis of HIV infection.
- Recovery applicants should be carefully screened to ensure that providers can ensure access to necessary and adequate medical care. Applicants who are so disabled by HIV infection that they cannot effectively participate in the activities or requirements of the setting in question should be referred for appropriate

medical attention and reconsidered for admission at a later date.

Federal, state, and many local laws prohibit discrimination against HIV-infected people in the provision of services, like alcohol or drug recovery, if the discrimination is based solely on HIV infection or an AIDS diagnosis. Most notably, the Americans with Disabilities Act, which became law in 1992, defines HIV disease as a disability and will protect disabled people from discrimination.

Local laws in many places, including New York, San Francisco, and Los Angeles, even prohibit discrimination against a person merely thought to be HIV-infected. These laws typically apply to both private and government-funded facilities and practitioners, but, in some jurisdictions, the stringency of enforcement may relate to the size of the facility based on the number of employees, number of clients, or amount of funding or income: the larger the provider, the greater the enforcement.

In addition, in most places, an institutional or individual practitioner may not discriminate against any prospective client who refuses to disclose HIV antibody status. A body of law developing in some southern states and Hawaii, however, may in the future allow practitioners to refuse service to clients who will not disclose antibody status. Under these circumstances, this "refusal to disclose" will not be considered a disability protected by discrimination statutes.

Unlawful discrimination can result in a lawsuit by an applicant against a recovery institution or provider. For instance, a 45-year-old alcoholic is rejected by a recovery program because he is HIV infected. Six months later, he dies. If his alcohol addiction was severe enough that his inability to obtain recovery services contributed to his death or a significant increase in medical harm to him, a court could award him or his estate a substantial amount of money in "damages." In addition, if while alive he complains to a state agency regulating alcohol and drug recovery providers, the agency may investigate and issue a violation notice against the program. If an alcohol or drug recovery program fails consistently to remedy discrimination violations, the state department could ultimately suspend the facility's license.

Substance abuse recovery programs, however, are not expected to treat medical conditions other than those relating to addiction and recovery. Indeed, program admission agreements, entered into with participants, should specify that the sole basis for admission is the detoxification and/or recovery of the participant. Recovery programs should make it clear to participants that the facilities are incapable of treating other serious medical conditions.

Similarly, individual recovery providers who have inadequate training in HIV-related mental health care may not be required to provide services beyond their area of expertise. The law, however, will not tolerate "patient dumping" or referral for HIV-related treatment when such referrals are made primarily in response to the program's or practitioner's fears of, or prejudices against, HIV-infected people.

Recovery programs or providers must refer for appropriate medical care those HIV-infected people whose immediate health conditions are so serious as to preclude them from effectively participating in a recovery program or plan. This sort of referral would not be considered discriminatory because it is in the best interests of the patient. In fact, a failure to make such a referral during the initial resident health screening or client interview might subject facilities to a state-issued deficiency notice or providers to malpractice claims.

Recovery providers should require applicants to identify serious medical problems, including HIV infection, during initial health screenings or interviews. This allows providers to make appropriate arrangements to ensure adequate medical, dental, and psychiatric referrals during the course of treatment or the recovery program.

2. Does a recovery program, or an individual provider, have to make special accommodations for the person with HIV infection? For example, must programs accommodate the use of prescription drugs or diminished physical condition?

- Providers should make appropriate accommodations for disabled people, including those with HIV infection, so that these people have adequate access to recovery programs.

- These accommodations are limited to those that do not defeat the overall treatment purposes of the recovery program.
- In general, infected participants should be maintained on their prescription drug therapies during recovery, so long as privacy is maintained, dosage and efficacy are monitored, and drugs are not used by staff and other participants.

Federal, state, and many local laws prohibit facilities, like alcohol and substance abuse recovery programs, from discriminating against people who are disabled or afflicted with certain medical conditions, including, for example, cancer and HIV disease. These laws have been interpreted by courts to mean that facilities must make "reasonable accommodations" to allow for nondiscriminatory access. For this reason, many such programs have, for example, wheelchair ramps and wheelchair-accessible toilet and bath facilities. The Americans with Disabilities Act adds further weight to these requirements.

These accommodations, however, will be deemed necessary only if they are required to afford access to participants and their necessity does not defeat the purpose of the program itself. For example, if one building at a recovery facility was accessible to a wheelchair and another building was not, the physically inconvenienced participant could not successfully argue that the program should go bankrupt renovating the other building simply because it had a better view.

To a lesser extent, these accessibility standards will come to apply to individual providers in the future. Depending on the size of the practice, its location, the costs and benefits of making it accessible, and the range of other accommodations that can be reasonably made to provide service to disabled clients, providers may be required to institute physical changes to meet the standards of the law.

Under these reasonable accommodation laws, HIV disease is no different from any other medical condition or disability. HIV-infected participants are entitled to the same access and respect as people with physical disabilities, including other medical conditions, and those with no disability at all. By failing to make the appropriate accommodations, recovery providers can be subject to lawsuits by

HIV-infected people or to investigations by state licensing agencies. Continued discrimination complaints could result in license revocations.

One accommodation that must sometimes be made is a reduction in work load for participants who, because of illness—for example, HIV disease, diabetes, or cancer—may not be capable of contributing as much physical labor as healthier participants. As long as other goals and objectives of recovery can be met, disabled residents must be excused from work they cannot do.

Of course, disabled participants who are disoriented or too incapacitated to meet the goals of the recovery program should be referred for medical assistance and not maintained in the program. As an aspect of recovery goals and objectives, this issue should be reviewed regularly to ensure both participation in the recovery program and maintenance of the health of participants.

Another accommodation, and one likely to be central to recovery programs, is the use of "licit" (legal) or health-sustaining pharmaceuticals by HIV-infected participants. In order to provide appropriate recovery services while maintaining the health and well-being of a participant, programs should generally allow participants to continue with prescription therapy, while frequently reassessing them for signs of addiction.

Indeed, without prescription pain killers, for example, some HIV-infected participants would be medically unable to function at a level sufficient to meet recovery program requirements. It may seem a contradiction—particularly among program staff and participants—to allow HIV-infected participants to "do drugs" while drug and alcohol use is not allowed in the facility, but, under the law, this accommodation must be made.

Treatment regimens must be charted in the health records of participants, and chart notes must include the name of prescribing physicians and instructions for the use of medications. Programs may require staff monitoring of prescription therapy, may insist that medications be taken in private away from other participants, and may require participants to maintain discretion about their medical regimen when interacting with other participants. Steps may be taken to ensure that HIV-infected participants do not "share" prescriptions with other participants or staff members, and sharing may result in expulsion or discharge of the HIV-infected participant.

In addition, after obtaining the written consent of participants, programs should regularly consult with participants' physicians to determine the efficacy of the treatment or pain-killer regime, proper dosages, and signs of addiction. If providers, participants, and participants' physicians determine that prescriptions or dosages, addiction, or the severity of untreated pain or other symptoms diminish the efficacy of recovery, treatment plans may be changed. It may also be appropriate to refer participants to facilities where program participation and medical treatment do not conflict.

Confidentiality

3. Do recovery programs have a right to know if participants are HIV antibody positive? May programs require antibody testing before admitting applicants? May individual providers require or request that clients take the antibody test?

- In general, providers have no "rights" to know the HIV antibody status of participants, but intake staff would be well-advised to attempt to sensitively obtain health status information from participants so providers can ensure adequate access to medical and other care during recovery. This information may be released to other providers or agencies only as allowed by law, in most cases only after obtaining the written consent of the participant to do so.
- Providers may not require HIV antibody testing of applicants as a condition of admission or care. This requirement is generally considered discriminatory and, in many states, opens providers to lawsuits or criminal prosecutions.

HIV antibody testing and confidentiality laws vary throughout the United States. A survey of laws from around the country indicates that providers are "safest" when they are most conservative, that is, restrictive, about disclosing HIV-related information. Providers should consult local AIDS legal service providers, disability rights programs, county counsels, or state attorneys general for more advice concerning specific local and state laws.

Requiring HIV antibody testing for applicants to gain access to alcohol or drug recovery programs is illegal discrimination in many states and locales. Nonetheless, it would be wise for providers to ask about antibody status or HIV diagnosis during the initial health screening or interview. This information might later be helpful to providers in ensuring that they can offer adequate medical and dental referral.

Participants, however, may not be forced to volunteer this information. During the process of eliciting this information, providers must explain to participants that this information will be used only to ensure appropriate medical care later. Unless participants give HIV-specific informed, and often written, consent to disclose antibody test results to recovery providers, providers have no "right" to know this information. Similarly, providers may not perform HIV antibody testing on participants without prior informed, and often written, consent. It is important to note that laws on this question, in particular, vary from state to state. (See also questions 4 and 5.)

Just as information concerning a participant's admission to a drug or alcohol recovery program is specifically protected by federal law, HIV antibody status (and, in some cases, other HIV-related test results) is generally protected by state and, often, local laws. Several state constitutions containing privacy protections may prohibit the disclosure of private or damaging information about a person, without the person's consent, even if this information is true. In most of these states, HIV-related information is considered private.

This privacy right is particularly significant for people with HIV disease. Many HIV-infected people have already lost their jobs, their homes, their children, their insurance, and their dignity because of the careless disclosure by others of HIV antibody status or AIDS diagnosis. Under many state constitutional privacy clauses, HIV-infected individuals may sue those responsible for disclosure, but such law suits cannot ultimately return to them what they have lost.

To further solidify privacy protections, most states have medical records confidentiality laws. These prohibit the disclosure by health care providers of any identifiable medical information on a patient unless the provider has that patient's prior written authorization. These laws often apply to substance abuse recovery facilities, other medical facilities, and individual mental health practitioners. Providers violating these laws may generally be sued for monetary damages, and in many cases may be subject to criminal penalties—in general, fines.

Finally, many states and localities have adopted specific legislation prohibiting the disclosure of HIV antibody test results (or other laboratory results indicating HIV infection) by anyone without the tested person's written or informed consent. In case of a later lawsuit against providers, it is still recommended that, even in those states requiring only informed consent for disclosure, that providers obtain written evidence of consent. Furthermore, in many jurisdictions, further written consent is necessary for providers to disclose antibody test results to additional people, unless disclosure is required as part of a government survey of the HIV epidemic.

Breaches of these legal standards may result in lawsuits against the recovery programs, staff members, or even private practitioners, and participants may request monetary damages, attorneys fees, and sometimes additional money as a punishment. If the breach is considered intentional, local prosecuting attorneys may also file criminal charges.

4. May counselors tell other providers that a participant is HIV antibody positive? May they tell other participants?

- Antibody test results, no matter how they are obtained, should not be disclosed by anyone to anyone without the prior informed, and preferably, written consent of the tested person.
- Providers may disclose this information without consent only when a health professional needs to know antibody status in order to provide appropriate diagnosis, care, or treatment to an infected participant.

Most states require prior informed consent before providers may disclose a participant's antibody status to anyone, regardless of how this information was originally obtained. For the best protection against litigation, this consent should be obtained in writing.

However, in some states there are exceptions that allow disclosure among certain licensed health care providers, for example, psychiatrists, psychologists, physicians, and psychiatric ward nurses. Under these exceptions, providers may disclose antibody test results without patient consent to other health care providers when disclosure is necessary for the diagnosis, care, or treatment of the patient or for the protection of a third party.

In the everyday routine of alcohol or drug recovery, these exceptions rarely, if ever, apply. The disclosure of antibody status might be necessary when a participant is to be referred to a doctor or hospital for HIV-related treatment because the information is obviously relevant to the diagnosis, care, or treatment of the patient. In most cases, however, antibody status should be carefully guarded.

Similarly, except in those narrow circumstances described below (see question 9 below), counselors should not disclose antibody status information about one participant to another participant without the first participant's consent. The disclosure of such information is likely to result in serious harm to the HIV-infected person, in terms of both discrimination and potential physical injury. This possibility—the disclosure and the resulting harm—should be reduced by frequent HIV-related education of participants and recovery staff and by dedicated protection of antibody information.

5. Do these guidelines change if a participant's medical provider, or someone else involved in his or her care, discloses this information to recovery providers? What if a participant's family member discloses this information?

- The guidelines for antibody test result disclosure remain the same no matter how the results were obtained.

Generally, laws protecting antibody test confidentiality do not change no matter who discloses the results. Sometimes, when a third party discloses antibody information about a participant, this disclosure is meant to incite discriminatory behavior against the participant. If providers further disclose this information negligently, a resulting lawsuit may attribute the discriminatory intent of the original disclosing party to the provider.

Whether or not the initial disclosure to a recovery provider was made legally or with discriminatory intent, redisclosure by the recovery provider is unlawful. Should harm result from this second disclosure, the recovery provider and program may be liable for large financial damages or penalties.

6. Can information about a participant's HIV antibody status be entered into his or her record? Can it be cited in provider notes?

- All information about a participant's antibody status should be charted in a special section of the participant's record.
- The information contained in that section should only be released when the participant gives HIV-specific, prior informed, and preferably, written consent for disclosure to a specifically named person or institution. In many states, even a subpoena requiring disclosure must be accompanied by an HIV- specific court order.

In most states, it is not considered an illegal disclosure of HIV antibody status for a health care provider to note antibody status in a patient's medical record. However, in many states and locales, antibody status—and the part of the record in which it is recorded—may not be further disclosed to anyone else without the patient's HIV-specific informed consent, in writing. Antibody status should, therefore, be kept in a separate section of the record that may not be shown to anyone without the patient's permission.

This same strict rule may apply to alcohol and drug recovery or community mental health program records. In fact, in some areas, like Los Angeles and San Francisco, alcohol and drug recovery program regulations prohibit the notation of any HIV-related information in the body of a participant's chart. All such information, even including notes that refer to a participant's fear of contracting HIV, must be contained in a "special section" in the back of the record. No one may gain access to this section without the written consent of the participant. Providers should check state and local laws to determine the stringency of local HIV-related regulations.

The purpose of these laws and regulations is to protect HIV-infected participants from discrimination and violence inside as well as outside of recovery programs. The most significant danger is that a participant's antibody status will be inadvertently disclosed to Medicaid, Medicare, or an insurance company that might then use the information against the participant, for example, by denying payment for a drug and alcohol recovery claim. It is always a tragedy when a participant, just beginning to get his or her life in order through alcohol recovery, loses his or her health insurance because of the recovery program's inappropriate disclosure of the individual's antibody status. To such a participant, alcohol recovery may not appear to have been such a good idea.

Duty to Warn and Permission to Warn

7. May providers inform a participant who has had some sort of unsafe contact with another participant—for example, through sexual activity or accidental blood exposure—that the other participant is HIV-infected? Must they disclose this information?

- Staff members do not generally have a duty to disclose HIV antibody status of participants to other participants or staff even if infected participants have engaged in behavior that might transmit HIV. Indeed, such a disclosure may violate the confidentiality of infected participants.
- Programs do, however, have a duty to educate staff and participants about HIV disease, "safer sex" behavior, and blood precautions so as to prevent the transmission of the virus. Mentally competent participants who still engage in unsafe behavior could be held liable for HIV transmission, and programs are within their rights to discharge such participants if this behavior is in violation of program rules.

The so-called "duty to warn" only applies to those licensed professionals, like psychologists, psychiatrists, and social workers, whose training and expertise equip them with the capacity to predict the possibility that their clients may engage in dangerous or threatening behaviors. The duty to warn generally does not apply to unlicensed recovery counselors because they have not had this special training.

Furthermore, the duty to warn (also called the "duty to protect") arises only when there is a genuine psychotherapist-patient relationship, when the patient communicates a serious and imminent threat of violence against another, and when the threat is directed at a reasonably identifiable victim or victims. If there was any threat in the situation described above, it was not a violent one (since the sex was presumably consensual and not rape) and even if the act had been violent, the threat had already passed, so it was not imminent. Therefore, there was probably no duty to warn.

However, some states have recently enacted criminal and civil statutes requiring people to inform health or law enforcement authorities about incidents involving possible HIV transmission between an infected person and someone else. In some states and in certain circumstances, this information must also be disclosed to the other person. Here again, providers should check with authorities to determine the local law.

In the absence of a duty to warn or a reporting statute, the program must maintain the confidentiality of HIV-infected participants. The only general exception to this rule, recognized in a few states, allows certain licensed health care providers, like physicians, to disclose the HIV antibody status of patients to the spouses, sex partners, or needle-sharing partners of these patients. Even in this circumstance, physicians are generally not required to make this disclosure, and this disclosure may be made only after physicians have tried to persuade patients to make the disclosures themselves.

One duty does arise in the scenario described above. The program and its counselors have a duty to appropriately supervise and educate program participants and staff members so that they are not subject to undue dangers. This duty would require appropriate AIDS awareness and "safer sex" education for both providers and participants.

Programs should emphasize the use of precautionary measures to avoid infection by the staff in handling blood or bloody situations. Similarly, participants should be correctly and thoroughly educated about the use of condoms and the avoidance of unsafe sex. They should be taught to ask, and honestly disclose when asked, about HIV infection status before engaging in sexual contact with other people. Recovery programs would also be well-advised to provide participants with condoms. After this initial education, staff members and participants alike should be counseled to assume that, when it comes to sex, needle sharing, and blood exchanges, they should assume that everyone is HIV-infected and should take appropriate precautions.

Finally, recovery programs should counsel HIV-infected participants that they should not engage in unsafe sex with other participants and that they should take appropriate precautions to avoid exposing others to blood. In these cases, providers should counsel participants potentially exposed to HIV about the risks and benefits of taking the antibody test. This counseling must not include disclosure of the identity of HIV-infected participants. Programs that fail to educate participants and staff members about HIV prevention or to appropriately counsel all parties involved in possible exposures could be sued for negligence by anyone who was inadvertently exposed to HIV while participating in or working at the program.

Once the provider and participant education has been done, participants and staff must assume the responsibilities to protect themselves and others from HIV transmission. For example, a participant knows that she is HIV-infected and still engages in unsafe sexual behavior with another participant without disclosing her infection status to that person. Under these circumstances, the partner could sue her if HIV is transmitted during intercourse. In some states, failure to disclose and protect can result in criminal liability—even prison sentences—to the infected person.

At the same time, sex partners, once appropriately educated by the program, have a duty to protect themselves from exposure, even if HIV-infected people do not disclose their status. Unless infected people lie about HIV infection status by denying it, their partners "assume the risk" of exposure when they engage in unsafe sex. Thus, as long as participants are mentally competent to understand about AIDS and safer sex, the primary duties to prevent HIV transmission remain with them.

8. If an HIV-infected participant has unsafe sex with someone who is not a participant in the recovery program, may providers inform the non-participant about his or her possible exposure to HIV?

- To protect non-participants facing possible HIV exposure after unsafe sex with infected participants, programs may inform non-participants about their potential risk of exposure but may not, in doing so, reveal the name of the participant. Public health departments usually provide this "partner notification" service.
- If the program has a well-explained rule prohibiting unsafe sex by participants, a violator may (and in some circumstances should) be expelled from the program.

Generally, providers may tell a non-participant that he or she might have been exposed to HIV, as long as providers do not violate the confidentiality of the infected participant. The most effective and anonymous method to do this is to contact the sexually transmitted disease tracing section of the local public health department. (In some states, this step may be required.)

Public health counselors are trained, in such situations, to provide appropriate information to the non-participant without violating the confidentiality of the participant. These counselors need not even inform the non-participant that the exposure might have been caused by a participant in the recovery program. This maintains the privacy of both the participant and the program, eliminating any liability to the program, while at the same time encouraging the non-participant to get tested for HIV infection and undergo available early intervention if necessary.

If the recovery program has a rule that prohibits unsafe sexual contact, and this rule is explained to participants as they enter the program and is accompanied by appropriate safer sex education, the violator of that rule may be dismissed from your program. In fact, to avoid liability to the program and to encourage safer sex by participants, such a rule, sanctioned by dismissal, may be necessary.

In addition, if a participant is recalcitrant in making safer sex behavior changes, poses a danger to multiple individuals through unsafe contacts, and is a threat to society as a whole, the therapist might consider another option. After warning the client that the therapist is about to take this step, the therapist could report the client to the public health department for its intervention under so-called "typhoid Mary" regulations. Under these laws, the health department may be authorized to investigate the situation, determine if the client is a danger to others, and then intervene, for instance, by holding the client for a period of time.

9. If a provider is in private practice, do duty to protect or permission to protect guidelines change?

- In general, duty to protect guidelines remain the same for providers in private practice.
- Certain psychotherapists and physicians may be required to warn or may be *relieved* of the requirement to warn depending on state law.

In general, providers in private practice must use the same analysis as recovery program personnel when determining whether they have a duty to protect. Licensed physicians, and licensed social work and psychological providers, however, have a stronger duty to protect than unlicensed employees of recovery programs. (See question 7 above for these guidelines.) Like agencies, these providers in private practice may also request public health department intervention in warning clients. (See question 8 above for a description of this process.)

In some states, certain psychotherapists and physicians may be required to report dangerous and recalcitrant clients to public health or criminal authorities under HIV-specific laws. In still other states, physicians and therapists may be required to report all cases of HIV infection to local authorities. Finally, in other states, physicians are *allowed* to disclose the HIV infection of their patients to the spouses, sexual partners, or injection drug partners of their patients, but, in most such states, physicians are *not required* to do this.

In these circumstances, the practitioner would be well-advised to contact a local AIDS law expert, the ethics committee of the practitioner's professional society, or the local health department before undergoing this kind of reporting. If such reporting violates a patient's right to privacy, his or her quality of life may be irrevocably affected.

Progressive Illness

10. If a recovery program participant is showing signs of HIV dementia (confusion, forgetfulness, difficulty thinking), is the program obligated to continue serving that participant? What if dementia progresses? May the program place the participant in another care facility?

- Alcohol and drug recovery programs are expected to provide recovery services only. They are not expected to provide medical care beyond that listed in their licenses. Participants in need of outside care must be identified as early as possible and referred to appropriate facilities.
- The possible need for medical care at some future date cannot be used to discriminate against HIV-infected participants. Infected participants should continue in recovery programs until completion or until their health conditions deteriorate to such an extent that they can no longer effectively participate.

HIV dementia results when the HIV disease process affects the brain and cognition, or thinking. A person with mild dementia may be forgetful on occasion. As the condition progresses, difficulties with speech, reasoning, and confusion are likely to develop. People with advanced dementia are unable to care for themselves: they may be confused about time, place, and person, unable to understand simple statements or commands, and incapable of communicating thoughts or wishes to others.

Alcohol and drug recovery programs are obligated to provide service only to those residents whose health conditions do not preclude them from effectively participating in the program. If HIV dementia or another psychiatric ailment—excluding alcohol or drug addiction, of course—or another medical condition is so severe as to make a participant unable to participate in recovery, that participant should be referred to an appropriate medical care facility for treatment. If and when the patient recovers from the ailment, he or she should be considered for readmission to the program.

Recovery programs are not generally expected to provide medical care beyond basic emergency first aid care. Programs that ineffectively provide such care could be subjected to a lawsuit for practicing medicine without a license or for negligence.

In this regard, it is important that all providers be effectively trained so that they can identify those participants who are suffering from health conditions requiring medical or dental care. Indeed, state laws generally require such training so that ill participants can be referred to appropriate care as quickly as possible. Similarly, the program must maintain a current list of appropriate consultants and health care providers so that referrals are effective.

The need for HIV-related treatment, however, may not be used as an excuse to discriminate against infected participants. These participants are as much in need of recovery services as are other people and should not be turned away from or moved out of a program just because they are infected. Illness, even some sign of dementia, is not automatically an indication that a person cannot benefit from a recovery program.

Harnessing the Law

While the law varies from location to location, its basic function remains the same: to protect the things society holds dear. For recovery providers, these elements may include: the recovery mission; recovery program participants or individual recovery clients; providers and their colleagues; the recovery program itself; and the greater recovery community.

In order to harness this protection, providers must be familiar with relevant laws and changes in these laws. Doing what he or she has "always done" may provide little protection in the face of changing laws and situations. And "following instructions" will not shelter individual providers if they have failed to consider the legal implications of their actions.

To ease their introduction to the law and their ongoing interactions with the legal system, providers would be well-advised to establish ongoing relationships with attorneys so they can answer legal questions as they arise. In addition, providers should consider having a lawyer perform a "legal audit" to gauge the state of compliance with the laws that govern program practice. Programs should then establish policies that facilitate provider compliance with laws and should offer legal training and updates.

All of this may seem difficult to grasp and overwhelming to accomplish, and providers may be tempted to let their legal obligations slide. But, although HIV-related law changes, basic tenets have been established, and these are easy to implement and ultimately protective of people in recovery and recovery programs.

References

1. Wood GJ, Marks R, Dilley JW. *AIDS Law for Mental Health Professionals (Updated Version)*. San Francisco: UCSF AIDS Health Project, 1992.

CHAPTER EIGHT

LOOKING AT POLICY

In This Chapter:

- Establishing HIV-Related Policies
- Intake Procedures
- Infection Control
- Confidentiality of Medical Information
- Medications for People with HIV Disease
- HIV-Related Training and Education
- HIV Antibody Testing for Participants
- Planning Policy Development
- Ethical and Philosophical Guidelines

CHAPTER EIGHT

LOOKING AT POLICY

ESTABLISHING HIV-RELATED POLICIES

Soon after I entered my recovery program, I told my counselor I was HIV infected. I wasn't exactly sure what I wanted from him, but I knew I was hoping for acceptance and understanding.

My counselor was supportive, and I knew he really cared about me and my situation. He also told me he hadn't had experience with people with HIV disease and this brought up some questions for him. I know he was confused, but as I look back on this, I can see that a couple of his comments were not very helpful.

First, he thought he might be obligated to tell his supervisor about my status, and he wanted my permission to do this. I agreed, even though I really didn't want anyone else to know about it just then.

Next, I asked if he could help schedule some kind of educational session about HIV infection for the program participants, because I had been hearing a lot of jokes and derogatory comments about AIDS. He said he didn't know how to do this as long as I wanted my circumstances to remain confidential. How could he explain why, out of the blue, the program was suddenly offering AIDS education to participants?

– Recovery Participant

Well-thought-out policies can help providers and participants alike, by setting forth guidelines that make appropriate actions clearer. HIV presents certain challenges in the matter of policy, but the epidemic does not raise new issues so much as it presses agencies to examine long-standing concerns. Properly crafted policies can help providers follow relevant laws, abide by ethical principles of their field of practice, and contribute productively to the overall mission of their agency.

Both administrative and line staff have significant investments in seeing that carefully crafted policies are developed and implemented in their programs. It is primarily the responsibility of administrators to evaluate the legal and ethical implications of policies. Administrators and line staff alike must consider whether policies are operational and functional in day-to-day practice. Are staff familiar with current policies? Are policies followed consistently? Do they contribute to the quality of service? Do they offer protections to staff or participants?

Policy questions are likely to arise as providers begin to offer HIV-related counseling and education. It would be most useful for providers to explore these sorts of questions before they are faced with HIV-infected participants. In planning such policies, there are several issues worth keeping in mind.

First, public attitude is more prejudicial toward HIV-infected people than toward people with other diseases. People with HIV disease often need additional, explicit protections concerning access to recovery programs and other services.

Second, concerns about medical treatment may arise for people with HIV disease, and these may complicate participation in recovery programs. For example, there may be questions about bed rest for individuals too ill to complete assigned chores in a recovery community or issues about the use of pain medications in an abstinence program.

Third, special counseling issues arise for people with HIV disease, those at risk, and people with friends who are ill. Policies need to be in place to support the education of staff on these issues and the provision of appropriate counseling.

Fourth, HIV disease has brought more attention to infection control in residential settings. To prevent HIV, hepatitis-B, and other blood-borne infections, standard infection control guidelines should be followed in all residential settings. In some agencies, these policies have not yet been established or implemented.

Fifth, HIV infection has raised special issues of confidentiality concerning medical conditions. Many policies need to be reworked and new policies written to address such issues. In some states, there are special laws concerning confidentiality of HIV-related test results. Providers need to be aware of such laws, and workplace policies need to be in compliance with them.

Sixth, there are HIV-related risks specific to people in recovery. HIV prevention education is an important facet of recovery programs and services. Policies about HIV education can help providers take the necessary steps to put such education in place.

Finally, to have the best chance of succeeding in recovery efforts, participants with HIV disease need support and acceptance from the recovery community. Policies encouraging education of all participants about HIV infection and related issues—for example, tolerance and acceptance, illness, death and dying, and health care—can establish a foundation upon which support and understanding are built.

In the following sections, a series of questions concerning policy are posed. These questions suggest points for reflection, and many are offered without specific answers. Each agency's situation is unique, and policies will need to be individually tailored to be most appropriate and effective; for a number of these questions, there are no "correct" answers. Commentaries in each section highlight further information relevant to the questions listed.

Intake Procedures

1. *Should there be a series of questions during intake that explore an applicant's HIV risk history?*
2. *Should there be a question about the applicant's HIV infection status? For example, has he or she taken the HIV antibody test and, if so, what were the results? Why might an agency want to know this information?*
3. *Should there be a standard intake procedure for all participants that reviews HIV-related risks and prevention, infection control guidelines, and resources for further information?*

Intake is generally the first contact between participant and program. At this delicate moment, it is essential that participants feel cared for and safe. Intake workers must be perceived as compassionate allies, not intrusive agents of an impersonal bureaucracy. At the same time, providers are obliged to gather a comprehensive range of personal information about participants so that adequate and appropriate care can be offered. Clear policy about intake procedures, along with careful training and ongoing supervision of workers, can help balance these sometimes contradictory needs.

In considering the above questions, several points are worth noting. First, responses to written, self-report questionnaires about HIV-related risk histories are often inaccurate. HIV providers recommend reviewing risk reduction information thoroughly and in person with all new participants at intake. They also suggest repeating this information at several points during the course of the program.

Additionally, specific questions about HIV infection status might be perceived by applicants as threatening. This would be especially true if such questions stood alone, rather than being part of a broader inquiry on medical status and history. Intakes may gather medical history relevant to the provision of care, however, and HIV infection might be one of the areas covered.

Intake procedures should be consistent for all participants, with information about medical history and health status requested on a voluntary basis. Providers must be careful when charting HIV infection status. Indiscriminate inclusion of HIV-related information in a participant's chart might violate state or local laws, or other program policies, even for uninfected individuals. (See also Chapter 7: *Legal Issues for Providers.*)

In many agencies, intake workers have limited training or experience. If basic HIV-related information and risk reduction guidelines are to be reviewed during intake, staff members will need comprehensive and ongoing training and supervision related to counseling about sexuality, injection drug use, death and illness, and other issues related to HIV infection.

Infection Control

1. *Is there a real or theoretical risk of HIV transmission in the workplace?*
2. *What guidelines need to be in place to prevent HIV transmission?*

3. *Do providers need different information about infection control than participants? Do providers need to follow different guidelines than participants?*
4. *How will providers and participants be educated about infection control procedures?*
5. *Who will be responsible for monitoring and enforcing infection control policies?*

Infection control appears to raise complex concerns. Of all HIV-related issues, however, infection control questions include some of the most straightforward, simple, and concrete responses. There are very specific guidelines, based on well-tested scientific principles, that can prevent transmission of HIV. Ambiguity stems not from the facts regarding HIV transmission and prevention, but from the personal anxiety people experience when they consider their risk for HIV disease.

There is little risk of HIV transmission in non-medical workplace settings. Nonetheless, familiarity and compliance with standard infection control guidelines will significantly diminish this already small risk. Agencies that need assistance in evaluating or developing infection control policies can check with local public health departments. Infection control experts are often available to offer consultation. (See also Appendix C: *Infection Control* for guidelines for residential and non-medical settings.)

Every member of a residential program, whether staff or participant, needs information about general infection control, and all should follow the same guidelines. These should be posted in a public place, such as the kitchen or a group meeting area. Providers may have additional responsibilities concerning infection control, for instance, in performing first aid or setting limits with participants who are not following guidelines.

Trainings on infection control should be provided for all staff, and repeated at regular intervals. Relevant guidelines and policies can be reviewed with new staff, as well as with new participants in residential programs. It is best if some kind of monitoring of infection control procedures is planned; without ongoing monitoring, infection control standards tend to become lax and are often neglected.

Confidentiality of Medical Information

1. *What medical information about participants do recovery providers need?*
2. *How should this information be gathered? For example, should it be based on the participant's self-report or on medical records from the participant's physician?*
3. *Who among the staff should be informed about a participant's medical conditions? Under what circumstances?*
4. *When is it appropriate, and who bears the responsibility for sharing medical information about a participant with designated staff?*
5. *What special policies need to be in place concerning records of a participant's HIV antibody status?*

Appropriate policies addressing the sharing and recording of medical information help protect the confidentiality of participants. This is often the central focus of concern when developing such policies. Another benefit, often overlooked, is that confidentiality policies also set guidelines that help providers resolve questions about clinical boundaries in their work. The policies clarify that it is not necessary for recovery providers to know all things about all participants in their program.

In general, staff should be informed of a participant's medical conditions on a "need to know" basis—that is, when the staff person would not be able to provide adequate care without that information. It may be necessary for a staff nurse or medical director to know of a participant's HIV disease, especially if the individual is symptomatic and needs medical follow-up. In most other instances, this information will be less essential to counselors or other staff members.

Federal, state, and local laws may regulate policies concerning charting or disclosure of HIV infection status. Agencies will need to be familiar with the laws relevant in their area and to their type of program. (See also Chapter 7: *Legal Issues for Providers* for further information, on confidentiality, charting, the "need to know" and relevant laws.)

Medications for People with HIV Disease

1. *Should a recovery program limit the use of HIV-related prescription medications among participants?*
2. *How are these medications to be stored? Who is responsible for monitoring the use of the medications: the participant, the participant's primary counselor, the program supervisor or a visiting or staff nurse?*
3. *Should there be policies concerning the education of staff on this matter? If so, how should these be structured?*

The issue of medications for the recovery participant with HIV disease or other chronic illness raises genuinely challenging questions for providers, especially in abstinence-based programs. Perspectives on this matter may vary from program to program; however, there are some essential guidelines to keep in mind.

Most importantly, the "Americans with Disabilities Act" (ADA) ensures certain rights of access for disabled people, including individuals with chronic illnesses. Limiting access to prescribed medications, as long as these are being used consistently with medical recommendations, is probably illegal under this law. Excluding people with chronic illnesses from recovery programs because they are using prescribed medications is also probably illegal.

If a program decides that a participant's medications will be stored and distributed by staff, the program would be well-advised to formalize this arrangement with the participant in writing as part of the recovery contract. Additionally, providers have an obligation to follow prescription guidelines in distributing the medications. (See also Chapter 7: *Legal Issues for Providers*.)

Providers and participants alike may feel conflicted when they try to understand how the use of prescription medications is integrated into a life without alcohol or other drugs. This is especially the case with medications that alter mood or thinking, which may be used by participants with advanced HIV disease. Staff trainings on this topic might include consultations among colleagues or with mentors, presentations by legal experts familiar with the provisions of the ADA, or clinically focused trainings by providers who have worked with individuals who use medications while in recovery.

HIV-Related Training and Education

1. *Should there be a policy supporting training for staff on HIV-related issues? If yes, whose responsibility should it be to develop and offer such trainings? How will the cost of trainings be handled?*
2. *Should there be a policy supporting education on HIV prevention for participants? If yes, whose responsibility should it be to develop and offer such education? How will related costs be handled? Should participants be given specific information about safer sex guidelines? Should they be given information about needle sharing and cleaning?*
3. *Should HIV-related education for staff and participants be ongoing or limited to a one-time workshop?*

Training and education are the absolute foundation for any success providers will have in stemming the spread of the HIV epidemic. These are also vehicles through which participants and staff alike can develop greater acceptance, understanding, and compassion for people with HIV disease. For these reasons, it is recommended that agencies have explicit policies supporting HIV-related training for staff, and HIV-related education for participants. In the absence of such policies, essential education may not take place.

People must hear information about HIV disease many times before they remember and understand it. Additionally, in most agencies, frequent changes among providers and participants makes ongoing training necessary. For participants in early recovery, the ability to comprehend and apply HIV-related information will improve as they become more comfortable and confident in recovery.

Finally, scheduling HIV-related education on an ongoing basis demonstrates a commitment to HIV prevention. This is important should providers or participants become HIV infected and should they claim that this occurred as a result of negligence on the part of the program.

HIV Antibody Testing for Participants

1. *Should the agency have a position either supporting or discouraging HIV antibody testing for participants?*

2. *Should HIV antibody testing be offered confidentially, on site?*
3. *If participants do choose to have an HIV antibody test, should anonymous testing be recommended over confidential testing?*
4. *If a participant does take the antibody test, should there be a policy discouraging that person from telling others about the test and results? Should there be a policy encouraging open discussion of testing and results? Should there be no policy on this matter?*

Policies concerning HIV antibody testing should be written so they do not contradict the law, but do protect the best interests of individual participants. In particular, special concerns for people in early recovery must be carefully considered in testing policy planning. All testing policies should support educated, informed decision making by participants. Finally, it is important to note that agencies providing on-site HIV antibody testing face significant challenges in maintaining confidentiality. (See also Appendix B: *HIV Antibody Testing.*)

Ethical and Philosophical Guidelines

1. *Should a special set of ethical and philosophical guidelines be developed concerning the agency's response to the HIV epidemic? For example, guidelines might include a clear statement supporting the participation of people with HIV disease—both participants and staff—in the recovery program.*
2. *If yes, what should the philosophical stance of the agency be? What ethical guidelines should be included?*
3. *If not, in what way should agency staff get an understanding of the agency's philosophy concerning HIV disease? Are there ethical principles or guidelines already set at the agency level that adequately address these issues?*

An ethical or philosophical framework can help provide a foundation for developing policies concerning HIV disease and other chronic illnesses. It can also be used to evaluate policy planning and implementation by asking, for example, whether a given policy is consistent with an agency's general position on people with HIV infection. Such tools can be useful in clarifying an agency's beliefs for both providers and participants. A statement specifically supporting the presence of people with HIV disease can increase the acceptance and comfort of HIV-infected individuals in a program.

Some providers feel that guidelines of this sort set HIV disease apart from other medical conditions, and confer a special status on people with HIV infection. This may seem undeserved or may appear to detract from the provision of appropriate service to all participants. However, providers should consider that the current social environment already distinguishes HIV infection as being more stigmatized and more broadly condemned than any other disease. Affirming the presence of people with HIV infection in recovery settings can serve to balance such attitudes.

Planning Policy Development

Proper planning and evaluation of policy involves a lot of time, research, and work. But good policies, actively implemented and supported by line staff, will ultimately save many hours and much distress, particularly when these issues arise during times of crisis.

For example, if an agency has already practiced standard infection control guidelines for some time, staff will be able to respond competently and appropriately should a person known to have HIV disease cut his or her hand, suffer a bout of vomiting and diarrhea related to food poisoning, or spit on the floor in an angry outburst. Providers who have benefitted from a policy encouraging staff trainings on HIV education and counseling will be able to support, for example, a participant who expresses despair about recovery after learning he or she has HIV disease.

Agencies that have a clearly stated policy of support for people with HIV disease seeking recovery will not create unnecessary obstacles for those who hit bottom and appear desperate and willing to stop drinking at any cost. And if other participants in a program complain about the presence of someone with HIV disease, clear policies will help providers respond appropriately and speedily, educating participants while supporting the HIV-infected person.

There is no question that HIV disease has complicated the work of recovery providers. By developing clear, relevant, and sound policy, providers can make much of this complicated material easier to handle. This necessary additional work will be rewarded, ultimately, with greater success in reaching participants and greater ease in helping them continue in their recovery process.

CHAPTER NINE

ACTION STEPS

In This Chapter:

- Taking The First Steps
- Why is It Necessary to Do Anything about HIV?
- Education and Support for All
- Develop Effective Counseling Skills
- Address Conflicts Raised by HIV Disease
- Helping People with HIV
- Helping the Recovery Community
- Where Do We Go from Here?

CHAPTER NINE

ACTION STEPS

Taking The First Steps

When the first person with AIDS came into our program, we didn't have a clue about it. We didn't know what it was, or how it could happen that alcoholics could get AIDS.

Looking back, we pretty much didn't want to know. It was easier then to say it wasn't our problem, and that we didn't have to do anything about it. We were happy to think that alcoholics were alcoholics, each one like the other, and that all they had to do was stop drinking, stay stopped, and the rest would follow.

Well, that's definitely the beginning. But there's so much more. It seems the norm these days for people addicted to alcohol to have drug addictions too. And addiction isn't the only killer disease people face.

Dealing with AIDS was a process. We had to think about so many things. It really helped when we realized that there was an organized way to approach these issues and the changes we had to make in our program.

Today, our staff knows a lot more about AIDS. We had to do some work to get there, but as a recovery home we've made room for this issue too. If our people have anything going on, we know helping them stay sober means helping them be honest and feel okay about it. Now, AIDS fits right in here.

– Recovery Home Counselor

The earlier chapters of this book show the many concerns that arise for recovery providers addressing the HIV epidemic. At times, the extent of these concerns may seem overwhelming. Where do providers get started? What kinds of actions can they take to keep momentum going once HIV disease is being addressed in their work settings? What are some approaches that can be used by individual providers, either in private practice or within agencies? What steps might be taken agency-wide?

Thankfully, there are also a number of straightforward actions providers can take. Many are quite simple and can be implemented by both sole providers and programs. This chapter outlines nine suggestions for providers and agencies responding to the HIV epidemic.

These suggestions range from educating participants about ways to avoid becoming infected with HIV, to sharing HIV-related information with colleagues, to simply listening and offering support to people with HIV disease.

For each suggestion, there is a series of action steps to implement the suggestion. Some are specific to individual providers, some to workplaces, and some to both. While it may not be practical to take every step listed, in most cases one or more steps will be possible.

(See also Appendix F: *Alcohol and AIDS Organizations* for suggestions about where to get information or educational materials, and Appendix D: *Participant Training Tools* and Appendix E: *Provider Training Tools* for materials that can be used to train staff and participants about HIV disease.)

Why is It Necessary to Do Anything about HIV?

HIV education is an essential element of recovery counseling for three reasons:

Facing the truth. The HIV epidemic poses challenges that are real and substantial. Many alcoholics have already been affected in some way by the epidemic, and others will be in the future. Twelve-step recovery encourages the practice of rigorous honesty, and recovery providers and agencies reflect this honesty when they are direct and truthful about HIV disease.

Supporting sobriety and recovery. An atmosphere of fear and doubt contributes little to a person's ongoing process of recovery.

By establishing an environment of acceptance and support, providers help participants maintain their commitment to recovery. When providers and workplaces directly face the challenges presented by HIV disease, they offer a working model of honesty, openness, and willingness that also reflects on broader recovery issues. If they neglect to do so, they may collude in a process of denial about the gravity of the HIV epidemic, raising conflicts and confusion for participants about HIV disease, specifically, and recovery, generally.

SUPPORTING HIV-INFECTED PEOPLE IN RECOVERY AND THE WELL-BEING OF THE LARGER RECOVERY COMMUNITY. Direct, honest, compassionate responses to the issues raised by the HIV epidemic also support the sobriety of people with HIV disease. Their success in recovery is more likely to occur in an environment that is supportive. Each individual's success contributes to the well-being of other alcoholics in recovery, to the well-being of their family members, and to the well-being of the larger recovery community.

EDUCATION AND SUPPORT FOR ALL

1. EDUCATE YOURSELF, COLLEAGUES, AND PARTICIPANTS ABOUT HIV DISEASE.

Information about HIV disease can save a person's life. It can also save an individual's sobriety.

The ability of providers to speak knowledgeably about HIV infection, and to respond to questions, can help build trust with participants. By educating participants and staff about HIV disease, workplaces can help people understand how serious the epidemic is. Education can also reassure people that there is no danger of casual transmission even when there are participants with HIV disease in residential programs.

ACTION STEPS:

- Stay informed about HIV disease. Attend HIV-related workshops at conferences. Talk to and learn from people with HIV infection.
- Put up HIV education posters in the office or agency. Post important news clippings about HIV disease on a bulletin board.

- Place educational pamphlets in the waiting area or community rooms.
- Have books about HIV disease available for loan.
- Provide staff trainings about HIV disease. (See also Appendix E: *Provider Training Tools* for suggestions and examples.)
- Provide HIV education sessions for participants. (See also Appendix D: *Participant Training Tools* for suggestions and examples.)
- Establish policies about HIV education that set standards for staff and participant education. (See Chapter 8: *Looking at Policy* for more suggestions about policy evaluation and development.)

2. Create an environment that welcomes ongoing discussion about HIV disease and related issues.

Most people have had little experience talking about sexuality, needle use, life and death, illness and disability, or homosexuality. But these subjects arise during discussions about HIV disease.

In early recovery, many participants do not know how to phrase questions about these matters. The actual words or language are unfamiliar; the questions are frightening; strong feelings, which are difficult to acknowledge, arise in response to these topics; or participants fear ridicule for raising such questions.

Providers help participants learn how to ask these questions by modeling open discussions about HIV infection and related issues. A willingness to have such discussions demonstrates that it is safe for people to ask questions and to get answers. Participants engaged in discussions about HIV disease feel supported when they state their concerns.

These discussions also offer an opportunity to repeat basic information about HIV prevention in an informal setting. Many people learn facts about HIV disease more easily in this way.

Action Steps

- Hang HIV education posters. Maintain a bulletin board with resource listings, prevention guidelines, and news clippings.

- Place educational pamphlets in waiting areas or community rooms.
- Demonstrate a willingness to engage in conversations about HIV disease. Initiate such discussions when the opportunity arises. Have these discussions in both one-on-one and group settings.

  Recent newspaper or magazine articles, or news reports on television, are good jumping-off points for HIV-related conversations. Or, a participant's comments about HIV disease, even if these comments are judgmental or negative in nature, may provide an opening for instructive discussion. For example, engage in discussion with a participant who says, "People with AIDS ought to be thrown out of this program."
- Provide staff trainings about HIV disease. (See also Appendix E: *Provider Training Tools* for suggestions and examples.)
- Provide HIV education sessions for participants. (See also Appendix D: *Participant Training Tools* for suggestions and examples.)
- Help participants learn to respect differences of opinion and perspective. Respond to incidents of teasing, hazing, racial or ethnic remarks, homophobia, or other personal attacks. Having a clear understanding about these issues will help create a safer environment for people to ask their questions and express their honest opinions about HIV infection.

3. Support people with HIV infection in exploring a 12-step approach to coping with their disease.

The 12-step model has been successful for people with a number of chronic, progressive, life-threatening diseases. It is useful for alcoholics, addicts, overeaters, and people who are codependent.

There is every reason to believe that this approach also helps people with HIV infection, also a chronic, progressive, life-threatening disease. There are many HIV-infected people who use a 12-step approach to help them cope with HIV disease. Some speak very powerfully of the strength and serenity they have gained from this application of the 12-step experience.

But just as a 12-step approach to alcoholism isn't the answer for every alcoholic, a 12-step approach to coping with HIV infection may not be the answer for every person with HIV disease. This will be true even if a person is participating in some other 12-step program of recovery. The Twelfth Step guides participants to practice the principles of the Twelve Steps in all their affairs. With this in mind, help participants understand 12-step resources and their options to apply them. Then, let participants decide for themselves what direction to take.

Action Steps

- Find out if there are HIV-related 12-step groups in your area. If there are, keep a current schedule of the groups handy. Share information about these groups with participants in a general way. For example, you may want to post a notice about the groups, including a contact telephone number. You may be able to get information about such groups by checking with a local AIDS information hot line, AIDS service organization, or gay community center.

  Remember that some people with HIV disease choose not to disclose their status. If you only give information about HIV-related 12-step groups to someone who asks for it, an individual who wishes to keep his or her HIV infection status private will not be able to get information about these groups.

- Study the ways the Twelve Steps apply to people with HIV disease. Read books or other resources that can help you understand more about HIV infection and the Twelve Steps. Read material on this subject, and talk to HIV-infected people who have used the Twelve Steps to cope with HIV disease.

- Develop an awareness of the ways in which concerns about HIV infection might affect sobriety or serenity. For example, someone who is very afraid of becoming infected is likely to be distracted by his or her anxiety. A person in new sobriety who learns he or she has HIV infection may find it difficult to feel hopeful about the future. A person whose sponsor is hospitalized with an HIV-related illness may feel frightened and confused.

Develop Effective Counseling Skills

4. Learn how to counsel participants about the HIV antibody test.

Some participants will want to consider taking the HIV antibody test. Some recovery programs directly encourage people to do so, however, many concerns arise for alcoholics taking the test. This is especially true in early sobriety.

Action Steps

- Become familiar with the HIV antibody test, including how it is performed and what its results mean. Understand the differences between anonymous and confidential antibody testing.
- Learn about the emotional reactions people in recovery are likely to have while considering taking the test, while waiting for results after taking the test, and after receiving results.
- Understand the pros and cons of taking the test, especially for people in early recovery.
- Read Appendix B: *HIV Antibody Testing* to gather further information about these and other issues surrounding HIV antibody testing for people in recovery.
- Identify the locations in your area where participants can receive either confidential or anonymous HIV antibody counseling and testing.

5. Establish ways to talk about sexuality with participants.

Sexuality is often a difficult issue for people in new recovery. Recovery providers have disagreed about what kinds of discussions about sexuality are appropriate. But with the advent of HIV infection, a life-threatening, sexually transmitted disease that currently has no cure, discussions about sexuality have become essential in recovery programs.

Action Steps

- Become informed on the human sexual response cycle, the range of human sexual expression, sexual health and HIV prevention, and sexual issues for alcoholics in recovery.

- Model comfort and acceptance in discussions of sexuality with participants. Provide opportunities for participants to discuss and consider their own issues regarding sexuality in sobriety.
- Pair discussions of sexuality and safer sex with clear, unambiguous messages about protecting sobriety and focusing on recovery.
- Have educational resources—brochures, books, and audio and videotapes—on sexuality, sexual health, and HIV prevention available for participants to take or borrow.
- Develop and offer a workshop series for participants on health issues, and include sexuality as one of the topics.
- Read Chapter 5: *Talking About Sexuality* to develop greater familiarity with issues which may arise when discussing sexuality and HIV with participants.

Address Conflicts Raised by HIV Disease

6. Support participants and providers in addressing the conflicts raised by HIV disease.

The HIV epidemic is not unique in presenting a series of difficult choices. Conflicts are a fact of life. Alcoholics, when they are drinking, typically avoid making conscious, straightforward decisions in the face of conflict. One of the tasks of sobriety is to learn to explore the choices presented and to take responsibility for dealing with them directly.

Clearly, a wide range of conflicts may arise when dealing with HIV-related issues in recovery settings. To be successful in HIV-related work, providers must expect such conflicts and be prepared for them. While the specific details of these conflicts may vary, some general responses will prepare providers to address them appropriately.

Some of the more common conflicts concerning HIV disease and alcoholics in recovery include:

Medication issues. People with HIV disease may require medications to treat symptoms or diminish pain. Abstinence programs must consider how to cope with a participant's use of such medications when these alter mood or thinking.

Full program participation. Providers must consider how they will respond to HIV-infected individuals whose limited physical energy precludes full participation in program activities.

Discussions of sexuality. It is essential to discuss sexuality openly and directly if providers are to succeed in HIV education efforts. These discussions can raise deep emotions, a sense of inadequacy in relation to limited experience or knowledge, or generalized anxiety. Providers must work to keep the focus on recovery within the context of these charged discussions.

Relapse issues. Alcoholism is a disease of relapse; it is not unusual for someone in early recovery to begin drinking again. A participant with HIV disease may well ask, "Why should I bother going through all of the pain and suffering of staying sober if I'm just going to die of AIDS?" Providers should consider what response they can offer this question.

General recovery issues. Traditionally, alcohol recovery programs have focused on maintaining sobriety above all else. Other personal issues are often set aside for some period of time so participants can keep their focus solely on recovery. This may not be advisable for a person with symptomatic HIV disease who needs medical treatment. The process of researching, seeking and obtaining care can be very time-consuming. There may also be a strong appeal to participants to become involved in community activism supporting HIV-related research or protesting government inaction. Providers will need to consider how to respond to participants in recovery, especially in early sobriety, who become deeply involved in HIV disease care or community activism.

Action Steps

- Acknowledge conflicts as they arise. Be willing to talk them over with participants. Discuss difficult issues with colleagues, seeking guidance from more experienced people and helping to educate those who are less informed.
- Validate the variety of experience colleagues and participants have. Acknowledge that opinions will vary. Keep the focus on supporting sobriety and recovery, and making the setting emotionally safe for people whether or not they have HIV disease.

- Explore some of these conflicts by raising them as topics in group meetings or staff trainings.
- Examine current policies as they relate to the issues outlined above, other conflicts that might arise, and general conflict resolution. Consider carefully whether policies need adaptation or amendment, or whether new policies need to be written.
- Read Chapter 5: *Talking About Sexuality,* Chapter 6: *Culture and Attitude,* Chapter 7: *Legal Issues for Providers,* and Chapter 8: *Looking at Policy* for more detailed discussions of issues likely to raise conflicts and suggested responses to these conflicts.

Helping People with HIV

7. Create a safe place for people with HIV disease.

People benefit from the acceptance and understanding of their recovery community. This helps them feel better about themselves and may help them maintain their sobriety. As basic as this suggestion sounds, this quality of acceptance for people with HIV disease is not always present in recovery settings.

There are people who continue to be afraid of "catching" HIV infection by being close to or touching people with HIV disease. There are others who are judgmental about HIV-infected people, believing that they must have done something wrong to get it. And there are people who discount individuals with HIV disease, because they believe the person will die soon and does not deserve or need attention or service.

People with these beliefs can be found in the recovery community, both as participants and providers. If they do not have an opportunity to educate themselves about HIV disease, they may never have the chance to develop opinions based on truth rather than conjecture. People with HIV infection will continue to suffer because of these misunderstandings and prejudices.

Action Steps

- Educate participants about HIV disease in a manner that establishes emotional safety for HIV-infected people. For example, new participants coming into programs should be educated about HIV transmission. This will include strategies to avoid infection, as well as clear information that HIV is not casually transmitted. Review the benefits of a compassionate and supportive attitude towards people generally, and with HIV disease specifically.

Providers can also be trained in these matters. In addition, they can speak with colleagues informally and engage in ongoing discussion about ways to create an emotionally safe environment for people with HIV disease.

- Emphasize to providers and participants that it is not useful to conceive of HIV infection as a fatal disease. HIV is a life-threatening, chronic, progressive disease. Treatments are available that can prolong health and well-being, and increase life span. Many people with HIV disease will live in good health for a decade or more, and as treatments improve, they live even longer.
- Model acceptance of people with HIV disease. If a person is publicly identified as having HIV infection, treat him or her the same as others participants. Shake hands, hug or speak individually with the person if these are usual behaviors. Let others learn by example. Be sure not to single out a person with HIV disease; for example, don't make a big deal out of hugging him or her if you don't usually hug others.
- Protect people with HIV disease by establishing proper infection control procedures and seeing that they are followed consistently. Most of the recommended steps in infection control help keep HIV-infected people safe from further infections. For example, regular cleaning of inside surfaces of refrigerators helps control molds that might pose a health problem for a person with HIV disease, although such molds would not harm a person with a healthy immune system. First aid policies consistent with universal precautions for handling blood should also be established and followed. (See also Appendix C: *Infection Control.*)

8. Help people with HIV disease learn self-advocacy skills.

People with HIV disease need to learn self-advocacy skills to deal successfully with the medical treatment system. They need to understand, for example, how to locate and utilize medical services, how to evaluate a physician's treatment recommendations, and where to go to learn about health or disability benefits.

Many of these steps will be difficult for a person in early recovery. They require assertiveness, persistence, and self-assurance. For their own well-being, HIV-infected participants will want to learn to take as much responsibility as possible for gathering information and making decisions about responding to HIV disease.

Providers may need to help alcoholics with HIV disease develop self-advocacy skills. This might include helping people see what options are available to them, helping them work out action plans for the options they choose to pursue, and modeling ways to deal with service providers. It is important that participants make their own choices about handling HIV disease. A useful guideline is, "Easy does it...but do it!" (See also Appendix B: *HIV Antibody Testing.*)

Action Steps

- Provide trainings for participants on self-advocacy and assertiveness skills. This might be done generally for a full group, or individually for a person with HIV disease.
- Maintain a good, up-to-date list of HIV-related referrals and resources. Identify HIV providers in the community who can help someone understand available resources, and make referrals to those providers as necessary.
- Facilitate finding HIV "sponsors"—other people with HIV disease, ideally people participating in recovery—for HIV-infected participants. This is especially relevant for people with HIV disease who do not have an identifiable community of support. The shared experience of talking with another person with HIV disease who is in recovery can be immensely valuable.

Helping the Recovery Community

9. Help maintain the trend of increased awareness, concern, and support for HIV-related issues in the recovery community.

The recovery community can contribute immeasurably to the well-being of HIV-infected people in recovery. To achieve this, providers and participants alike will need to keep HIV-related issues in mind, but this work is not "completed" simply by having a good general understanding of these issues. Providers must continue to learn from people with HIV disease and to reach out with support to them. Providers must also acknowledge and appreciate their own HIV-related issues and risks.

There is a resistance among some participants and providers to the idea that HIV disease—and its related risks—is a relevant issue for alcoholics. People may deny the extent to which polydrug use exists among individuals whose drug of choice is alcohol. In some settings, there seems to be a greater acceptability of the "pure disease of alcoholism," over the disease of drug addiction or polydrug abuse. It is a simple matter of fact, however, that many alcoholics have also used other drugs, including injection drugs, and may risk HIV transmission in this way.

There may also be a resistance to seeing that risks of sexual transmission exist for some alcoholics. The fact is that alcoholics, like other people, may have engaged in sexual activities that have put them at risk for HIV infection. This is true for men and women. It is true for people who are heterosexual, bisexual, lesbian, or gay.

A person struggling with fears of death, uncertainty about the future, anger at an insensitive doctor, or frustration at a new physical symptom, may need to talk about HIV disease in order to stay sober. Sometimes, however, people who speak at AA meetings about having HIV disease have been told this is not an appropriate topic for the meeting, that the focus should be on working the steps and maintaining sobriety. It may be difficult to determine whether someone with greater experience is helping a person stay focused on their program or expressing personal anxiety about people with HIV disease, in general, or gay people, needle users, or other people identified with the epidemic.

There are also people with HIV disease who have disclosed this fact at a meeting, and later found that their anonymity had been violated. In one instance, for example, individuals who were not present when a person spoke about having HIV infection approached him later with words of sympathy and concern. They meant to lend support, but only enforced that his anonymity had been broken. Providers and participants alike must work to create an environment where anonymity— about alcoholism, HIV disease, marital problems, job dissatisfactions, or anything else—is respected.

Action Steps

- Support the scheduling of HIV-related topics at conferences and meetings.
- Support a person with HIV disease who chooses to attend a gay AA meeting, or an HIV-specific AA or 12-step meeting. This may be an excellent opportunity for that individual to combine program recovery and HIV-related recovery in an appropriate and supportive setting.
- Discuss with colleagues the general issues of how to best support participants who are affected by HIV disease. Acknowledge the conflicts, and talk about some of the difficult issues such as anonymity and staying focused on sobriety.
- Model acceptance and support for people with HIV disease. Always maintain the anonymity of HIV-infected people.
- Establish and maintain appropriate policies and practices concerning confidentiality of medical information, including HIV infection status.

Where Do We Go from Here?

Perhaps the greatest danger in responding to the HIV epidemic is developing a sense of complacency—"We've done all we need to do,"—or indulging the feeling that there is nothing that can be done at all. The suggestions in this chapter demonstrate that there is much that every recovery provider can do. By taking some of these action steps, providers can make progress in two goals: to educate participants and colleagues about how HIV disease is, and is not, transmitted, so they can protect themselves from infection; and to provide support for people with HIV disease, to help them maintain sobriety, and physical and spiritual well being.

This book has covered a lot of information and has offered numerous suggestions to help alcohol recovery providers reach these goals. The HIV epidemic is many-faceted, can be overwhelming, and places complicated demands on all kinds of service providers, particularly in the field of recovery work.

One of the tendencies providers must guard against is the feeling that all of this is too much to do, too difficult to understand, too hard to remember. As is so often the case, some tools of the 12-step program may be useful to keep in mind.

KEEP IT SIMPLE. No one needs to learn all of the information in this book at once, or implement all of the suggestions immediately. Bringing HIV-related counseling and education to the recovery setting is a task that demands sensitivity and skill, and it will take time for providers to find ways to integrate the information into their work. But by doing a little bit every day, it is possible to build the groundwork for change and to see change happen.

TALK TO EACH OTHER AND REASON THINGS OUT. Don't try to do all of this work by yourself. In order to reach an understanding of how to support people coping with HIV-related issues while in recovery, talk with friends and colleagues, mentors and advisors. By sharing thoughts with others, we can find wisdom and experience that reaches beyond what we know as individuals. Solutions to many problems become simple and clear with such insights.

LET UNDERSTANDING AND PEACE GROW, LITTLE BY LITTLE. HIV-related counseling and education can be hard work. But as understanding grows, so does confidence and acceptance. With experience, you will be clearer about what you can do to help participants, and what you cannot or should not do. With practice, little by little, HIV-related work will become almost second nature. When providers can offer this support to participants, to friends, and to colleagues affected by the epidemic, the recovery community itself will become stronger, and the fight against the spread of HIV disease will be strengthened as well.

APPENDICES

In This Section:

APPENDIX A

OVERVIEW OF ALCOHOLICS ANONYMOUS

THE HISTORY OF ALCOHOLICS ANONYMOUS

Alcoholics Anonymous (AA) was founded in 1935 by two alcoholics, Bill W. and Dr. Bob. These men had tried all the approaches common at that time to cure their addiction to drink, but each found himself repeatedly sobering up, then drinking again. Their health, their careers, and their families were in chaos, and Bill W. and Dr. Bob were desperate for help. They were willing to go to any lengths to succeed in their goal of achieving sobriety. It was out of this tremendous desperation that the Twelve Step program of Alcoholics Anonymous was born.

The founders based AA on three premises. First, alcoholism is a disease: alcoholism has specific and predictable physiologic effects, it is progressive in nature, and its progression continues as long as an individual continues drinking. Alcoholics neither choose to be so afflicted, nor are they able to control the powerful compulsion to drink.

Second, one alcoholic can talk to another with an impact that no non-alcoholic can ever achieve. The shared experience of alcoholics contributes to the ability of individual alcoholics to recognize, and then address, their alcoholism.

Finally, conscious contact with a "higher power"—a power greater than oneself—is essential to living without alcohol. Alcoholics are unable to control the course of their disease or stop drinking on their own. With a spiritual program, it becomes possible for them to do so.

These three premises suggested to Bill W. and Dr. Bob the program of "Awareness, Acceptance and Action" that is outlined in the Twelve Steps.

About the Twelve Steps

At the First Step, the alcoholic admits being powerless over alcohol. This is a concept that confuses many people unfamiliar with the AA program. "How can people be empowered to change when you are telling them they are powerless? What use is 'powerlessness' to someone who is already disenfranchised or depressed, or suffering the effects of homelessness, classism, racism, or sexism?"

But, in truth, alcoholics *are* powerless over their alcoholism. It is a fact of life—much like having brown eyes or growing up in New York City.

Alcoholics can try to control their drinking, deny having a problem with alcohol, or claim to be unaffected by the physical and social consequences of drinking. These attempts to manage alcoholism lead to misplaced and fruitless efforts. AA's First Step offers a chance to let go of that pointless struggle. The alcoholic is an alcoholic. An alcoholic is powerless over alcohol. Efforts to manage drinking are doomed to failure. Once an alcoholic becomes "aware" of this, it is possible to direct his or her energies to more productive endeavors.

The Second Step of AA describes a "Power greater than ourselves" that can assist the alcoholic in staying sober. This higher power might be a religious figure, such as God; but for alcoholics who do not believe in God, the higher power can be the group of alcoholics who attend AA meetings ("Group Of Drunks = GOD"); the Twelve Steps of AA or other principles or traditions of the program; or a sense of some universal consciousness, fate, or wisdom. AA makes no demand on the type of higher power an alcoholic chooses. The program only asks that the alcoholic "accept" the existence of some power greater than him or herself.

In the Third Step, the alcoholic makes a decision to turn his or her life over to the care of this higher power. This is the first "action" step of AA. The Third Step reassures the alcoholic embarking on the difficult and challenging path of recovery that he or she will be cared for in this process.

The remainder of the Twelve Steps outlines the course of continued action alcoholics can follow to pursue recovery. Sobriety is never guaranteed. It can only be achieved by practicing the principles of the AA program one day at a time.

About the Twelve Traditions

The Twelve Steps guide the individual through recovery. AA's Twelve Traditions offer guidance at the group level, providing suggestions that maintain the integrity of each AA group and the larger AA fellowship. Without the Traditions, individual personalities might divert AA from its primary purpose—to carry its message to alcoholics who still suffer. When AA members abide by the Traditions, their own recovery processes are strengthened.

Among the suggestions included in the Traditions are:

Requirements for membership. The only requirement for membership in AA is a desire to stop drinking.

Free program. AA is a free program, supported entirely by voluntary member contributions. Each AA group is fully self-supporting. AA declines all outside contributions.

Outside issues and endorsements. AA takes no opinion on outside issues, avoids controversy, and offers no endorsements. Its sole purpose is to provide assistance to alcoholics.

Anonymity. Anonymity is the foundation of the AA program. This protects the privacy of the alcoholic, and keeps the focus on the principles of the program rather than on the personalities of individual members. Members are advised to maintain personal anonymity in interactions with the news media.

Additional Key AA Program Elements

Other key concepts of AA are outlined in additional program literature. Knowledge of a few will be especially useful for providers.

Sponsorship. New members are encouraged to establish a relationship with a "sponsor," often a person with more time in AA and more experience in recovery. Sponsors can support alcoholics by offering their own experiences in using the program tools.

SPIRITUALITY. AA is a spiritual program based on no particular form of religion. It is not affiliated or allied with any sect or denomination.

SERENITY. Serenity is possible for the alcoholic in recovery who is able to accept those things that cannot be changed, change those things which can and should be changed, and knows the difference between the two.

INDIVIDUALITY. Some people unfamiliar with AA worry that it is a cult. Cults, by definition, minimize individual differences and try to disempower members. AA, on the other hand, emphasizes the individuality of each alcoholic's program of recovery. "Take what you like, and leave the rest," members are advised.

There is a shared language among AA members, and the program itself represents a common solution to the problem of alcoholism. But people of all political and professional affiliations, religions, nationalities, genders, sexual orientations, ages, races, and classes, have been able to apply the principles of AA to their lives, without in any way sacrificing these other affiliations or identities.

THE TEXT OF THE TWELVE STEPS*

1. We admitted we were powerless over alcohol—that our lives had become unmanageable.

2. Came to believe that a Power greater than ourselves could restore us to sanity.

3. Made a decision to turn our will and our lives over to the care of God *as we understood Him.*

4. Made a searching and fearless moral inventory of ourselves.

---

*The Twelve Steps and the Twelve Traditions are reprinted with permission of Alcoholics Anonymous World Services, Inc. Permission to reprint the Twelve Steps does not mean that AA has reviewed or approved the contents of this publication, nor that AA agrees with the views expressed herein. AA is a program of recovery from alcoholism—use of the Twelve Steps in connection with programs and activities which are patterned after AA, but which address other problems, does not imply otherwise.

5. Admitted to God, to ourselves and to another human being the exact nature of our wrongs.

6. Were entirely ready to have God remove all these defects of character.

7. Humbly asked Him to remove our shortcomings.

8. Made a list of all persons we had harmed, and became willing to make amends to them all.

9. Made direct amends to such people wherever possible, except when to do so would injure them or others.

10. Continued to take personal inventory and when we were wrong promptly admitted it.

11. Sought through prayer and meditation to improve our conscious contact with God, *as we understood Him,* praying only for knowledge of His will for us and the power to carry that out.

12. Having had a spiritual awakening as the result of these steps, we tried to carry this message to alcoholics, and to practice these principles in all our affairs.

The Text of the Twelve Traditions

1. Our common welfare should come first; personal recovery depends on AA unity.

2. For our group purpose there is but one ultimate authority—a loving God as He may express Himself in our group conscience. Our leaders are but trusted servants; they do not govern.

3. The only requirement for AA membership is the desire to stop drinking.

4. Each group should be autonomous except in matters affecting other groups or AA as a whole.

5. Each group has but one primary purpose—to carry its message to the alcoholic who still suffers.

6. An AA group ought never endorse, finance, or lend the AA name to any related facility or outside enterprise, lest problems of money, property or prestige divert us from our primary purpose.

7. Every AA group ought to be fully self-supporting, declining outside contributions.

8. AA should remain forever nonprofessional, but our service centers may employ special workers.

9. AA, as such, ought never be organized; but we may create service boards or committees directly responsible to those who they serve.

10. AA has no opinion on outside issues; hence the AA name ought never be drawn into public controversy.

11. Our public relations policy is based on attraction rather than promotion; we need always maintain personal anonymity at the level of press, radio and films.

12. Anonymity is the spiritual foundation of all our Traditions, ever reminding us to place principles before personalities.

APPENDIX B

HIV ANTIBODY TESTING

The HIV antibody test is a simple blood test that can determine whether or not an individual is infected with HIV. The information provided by the test can be useful in many ways. A person who learns he or she is not infected may be motivated to practice HIV prevention guidelines and avoid exposure to the virus in the future. A person who learns he or she does have HIV infection can avoid passing the virus to others and seek medical treatment to maintain better health.

The role of the antibody test for people in recovery, especially in early sobriety, is complex. Providers differ about whether the test is appropriate, necessary, and useful for such individuals. In early recovery, when an individual's decision-making skills may be limited, deciding whether or not to be tested can be especially challenging. Providers working with people in recovery may be asked to assist in this process by providing information, support, and guidance.

This appendix reviews background information about the test, describes the process of antibody testing, and covers related issues, including the special concerns of HIV antibody testing for people in recovery. In the future, new methods for testing for HIV infection may become available. In this event, much of the information in this appendix will remain relevant.

The HIV Antibody Test

The human immune system responds to HIV much as it does to other viruses. A few weeks or months after a person is infected, the immune system develops antibodies—specialized proteins to help fight a particular infection. These antibodies circulate in the blood. When they identify the virus, they attempt to destroy it. The antibodies to HIV seem to help slow the progression of the disease, but they are not able to completely eradicate the virus. Over time, most people develop HIV-related illnesses.

Antibodies to HIV can be detected with the help of a blood test called the *HIV antibody test*. To perform the test, a couple of tablespoons of blood are drawn, the test is run on the blood sample, and a week or two later, the results are available. The results will either be *positive* (HIV antibody was found in the blood), or *negative* (no HIV antibody was found).

The test for HIV infection looks for antibodies rather than the virus itself, because the antibody test is cheaper, easier to perform, and more accurate than the test for the virus.

What Do These Results Mean?

Negative test result

A negative HIV antibody test result indicates that no antibody was found in the blood sample. One of the following is true: the person has not been infected with HIV; or the person has been infected with HIV, but has not yet developed antibodies. It may take anywhere from two weeks to six months for a person infected with HIV to develop antibodies. This means it is possible in some cases for a person who tests negative on the antibody test to be infected with HIV.

How might this happen? Imagine that a woman requests an HIV antibody test because her sexual partner has used injection drugs. If her last unsafe sexual contact with her partner was two weeks ago, she might have become infected at that time. However, antibodies to the virus might not have developed during this two week period. In this case, she would have HIV infection, but her antibody test would be negative, indicating that no antibody was found in the blood sample.

If she were tested and if her first test was negative, it would be important for this woman to return in about six months for a second antibody test. If the second antibody test was also negative, and the woman had not engaged in any HIV-related risk behaviors during that time, she could be fairly confident that she was not infected with HIV.

In a few cases, individuals have been infected with HIV and have not developed antibodies for two years or more. Extensive investigation into this matter has shown it to be a rare occurrence. The vast majority of HIV infected individuals will develop antibodies within six months of infection.

Positive test result

A positive test result indicates that an individual is infected with HIV and has produced antibodies to the virus. He or she is also capable of passing the virus to others during unprotected sexual intercourse or needle sharing. A positive antibody test result does not offer information about the health of the immune system or how far HIV infection has progressed.

People who test HIV antibody positive should plan to see a physician familiar with HIV disease soon after receiving test results. Other tests can provide information about the status of the immune system. Based on the results of these tests, the physician may recommend the use of medications to slow the progression of the disease and regular visits to monitor the immune system.

Indeterminate results

In rare cases, a test result is neither clearly positive nor clearly negative. In these instances of "indeterminate results," blood is usually redrawn and the test is performed again. Generally, the second blood sample will provide a clear result.

HIV Antibody Test Counseling

Counseling is an essential part of the antibody testing process. Before blood is drawn for the test, a trained counselor should provide "pre-test counseling." This counseling includes a description of the testing procedure, an explanation of what the test results mean, an assessment of HIV-related risk, and HIV prevention education. This information is particularly important in light of the legal requirements in most states that HIV antibody testing be performed only with a client's informed consent. Providers also have an ethical obligation to promote the welfare of participants and clients, and this includes the assurance that clients understand and willingly choose to have an antibody test. Finally, pre-test counseling provides an opportunity for clients to discuss related concerns in a private setting.

One-on-one counseling is the preferred model for pre-test counseling, although in some settings it has been necessary to provide group education sessions to cut costs. Ideally, an individual seeking testing will have an opportunity for some one-on-one contact with a counselor to ask personal or sensitive questions.

When test results are available, they should be given to the individual during "post-test counseling." One-on-one counseling is the only model that should be used in these sessions. Again, a trained counselor should provide the test results, help the client understand the meaning of the results, and assist the client in preparing a health plan for the future. Whether the individual tests positive or negative, the counseling should cover HIV risk reduction—how the person can avoid behaviors that might put him or her or others at risk for HIV infection or reinfection. Those who test antibody positive should be encouraged to seek knowledgeable medical care; support from family, friends, or others; and counseling, support groups, benefits counseling, and other referrals if appropriate.

HIV antibody test counseling should always be provided in person. The results, whether positive or negative, should be discussed carefully with the client as this sensitive information is likely to raise powerful emotions. It is not appropriate to discuss such matters by telephone, recorded message or letter.

Anonymous versus Confidential Testing

HIV antibody test results must remain private. There are two strategies that have been developed to achieve this.

The first is "anonymous" testing. Individuals being tested are identified only by a code number, which they must present to receive their test results. Counselors do not know clients' names and cannot locate or contact clients for any reason. When clients give informed consent to be tested, they do so verbally; no signature is required to take the test. There is absolutely no way to link a person's test result with his or her identification, and no third party can ever receive the results.

The other strategy, "confidential" testing, is based on the medical model of confidentiality. Confidential testing is usually performed through medical clinics or private medical offices, and may be performed in drug treatment or other facilities. Clients are identified by name, and informed consent is written. Test results will usually be recorded in the medical record. They cannot be released, except as allowed by law, and this usually requires written consent.

There are pros and cons to both styles of testing. The benefit of anonymous testing is the absolute privacy of test results. No one can know the result unless the person tested chooses to disclose the information. There are no medical records of the test that can be released to any provider, agency, or insurance company. There can be no unauthorized breaches of the records because no records linking the person's name and his or her test result exist.

But to be truly anonymous, a client should be counseled by someone who does not know him or her. As a result, the counselor will not be aware of the client's longer term health concerns or special issues unless the client discloses these during the session. To maintain anonymity, the counselor is usually not able to offer personal follow-up to the client, but must rely instead on referral to other providers. There is no way to check back with the client to see if referrals were followed, whether they worked out, and whether the antibody positive client has seen a physician.

Confidential testing enables the counselor to be familiar with the client's medical records and may facilitate follow-up appointments to address HIV-related issues. This capability can be especially helpful for people who are in vulnerable emotional states—perhaps including people in early recovery—and who might have an unusually difficult time coping with the waiting period for test results or with the test result itself.

The drawback—and it is a significant one—is that after confidential testing, there will be a medical record that links a person's name with the fact he or she took the test and with test results. Intentional and accidental breaches of confidentiality could result in discrimination, the loss of employment, and the loss of insurance coverage.

Anonymity in Small Communities

In some settings, true anonymity may be virtually impossible. For example, at smaller, rural test sites, a counselor and client may know one another personally. While no written connection between the client and his or her results is made, the counselor will be aware of the client's test result. Legal guidelines prohibit the disclosure of that information to any third party, but the fact remains that disclosure by oversight or negligence is possible. In other kinds of "small communities"—residential recovery programs, for example—true anonymity may also be impossible to establish. At sites where anonymous testing is offered, clients may be identified by community members simply by their presence in the waiting area.

The actual results of the antibody test are sometimes obvious to observers as well. If counselors provide shorter post-test counseling sessions to individuals who test negative, and longer sessions to those who test positive, anyone aware of the length of the session can guess the likely results.

There are solutions to these problems. Individuals in rural communities often travel to other regions to be tested so anonymity is protected. Small recovery or service agencies can avoid offering anonymous testing on-site. Where anonymous testing is the preferred choice, refer participants to outside agencies. Private waiting areas may be available for people waiting for counseling and testing.

Responding to a Positive Result

Usually, receiving a positive HIV test result is a difficult and frightening experience. Many people assume it to be a "death sentence," a hopeless diagnosis. Panic, confusion, and despair are common reactions. It is not unusual for individuals who have been given a positive test result to have suicidal thoughts and feelings, or to imagine that life is over.

While HIV infection is a serious, life-threatening disease, it is essential to understand that many HIV-infected people are doing very well after several years of infection. Today, a number of medical treatments are available for people with HIV disease. These treatments may extend a person's health and life span by limiting the replication of the virus and slowing the progression of the disease. There are also medications that help prevent the onset of common, HIV-associated diseases, as well as treatments that can successfully resolve some of these illnesses if they do develop.

A useful message for people who test positive is one of realism and hope. Yes, this is a serious disease. It will be important for the participant to take steps to protect his or her health and promote physical and emotional well-being. But there is also reason to be hopeful: hopeful that treatments currently available can help people stay healthy and energetic; hopeful that new drugs being developed will be more successful in fighting the disease; and hopeful that in the not-too-distant future, HIV infection will become a manageable disease in the same way diabetes is today.

Deciding Whether to Take the Test

Participants should be encouraged to think carefully about antibody testing and helped to understand the pros and cons of taking the test. Medical experts believe that testing is a wise idea. Treatments are now available for individuals with HIV infection and are sometimes recommended even if a person feels healthy. Determining HIV antibody status and, further, immune system status, is the first step to protecting health.

On the other hand, individuals in recovery are already involved in a program designed to address the life-threatening disease of alcoholism. The challenges of this recovery process are considerable. In exploring questions about the antibody test, participants will want to consider what they would do if test results were antibody positive. Would this present a challenge to sobriety? Could it precipitate a slip? Participants must weigh the risks and benefits of testing and consider not taking the test—"just for today"—realizing that they may make a different decision in the future.

There are no absolute answers or recommendations for people in recovery concerning the antibody test. This is a deeply personal decision that participants must make for themselves. It is clear that participants must have adequate support in place to address alcoholism before they can competently address other life issues, including other life-threatening medical concerns. Taking action concerning antibody status should be part of the overall healing process in recovery, not an invitation to slip.

In some recovery settings, providers find themselves acting as decision-makers for newly sober participants. A recovery counselor may structure a participant's daily routine, indicate which meetings he or she should attend, evaluate what pastimes are acceptable, and decide which friends the participant should visit. When participants need to focus all of their energy on maintaining their sobriety, a day at a time, this help in making decisions can be useful and appreciated.

In the matter of antibody testing, however, it is essential that individuals make their own decisions. If participants are incapable of making decisions about testing, the decision process should be delayed until they are able to do so.

Recovery seeks to promote health, prolong life span, and improve the quality of physical, emotional, and spiritual life—to help alcoholics learn to live with this chronic, life-threatening illness. Similarly, HIV antibody testing can offer opportunities for people who have HIV disease to live healthier, better, and longer lives. Unlike recovery, however, where stopping drinking is the necessary first step, there is no "right" answer regarding HIV antibody testing. Counselors must support participants in their own process to discover the right decision for themselves.

Rigorous Honesty: Being Fearless and Thorough

Alcohol recovery demands rigorous honesty in all one's affairs. Participants are repeatedly reminded to be fearless and thorough in examining their recovery as well as other aspects of their daily lives.

HIV disease, however, presents a dilemma in this light. When a participant discusses personal concerns about HIV disease, some people may respond with fear or judgment. They may be unable or unwilling to honor the confidentiality of such matters. When is it helpful and appropriate for a participant to talk openly about taking the antibody test or receiving results? When might it be appropriate to keep such information private? Participants are encouraged to "carry no secrets" in their recovery; when could it be harmful either to disclose, or to withhold, this kind of information?

Once again, there can be no absolute answers to these questions. It is helpful, however, to discuss the matter of rigorous honesty with participants and to emphasize that this does not require full disclosure of all personal information to everyone in the program. Recovery participants often need help learning about appropriate boundaries, and HIV-related issues can offer an excellent example of this principle.

In some instances, choosing not to share HIV-related information might be the wisest course of action. Participants do not benefit from asking other individuals in recovery to give more than they are capable of giving. If people are frightened or judgmental about HIV-related issues, the HIV-infected participants may not get the support they need at an emotionally fragile and potentially slippery time.

On the other hand, secrets that threaten sobriety do pose a danger to the alcoholic in recovery, and it is in these areas that rigorous honesty is essential. For example, if a health crisis is frightening a participant and making him or her think about drinking, it is important to share this within the group. It is not essential to share the specific nature of the health crisis, for example, HIV disease, hepatitis, or cancer. Or a participant obsessing about past behaviors that might have put him or her at risk for a serious disease may fantasize that a drink would relieve this obsession. The participant can discuss these thoughts and feelings without describing specific past behaviors or the particular disease.

Who Needs to Know a Participant's HIV Antibody Status?

Recovery providers may themselves face challenging issues in the area of HIV-related disclosure. They may want to be familiar with issues of emotional importance to participants. Concerns about HIV-related risks or knowledge that one is HIV antibody positive certainly seem to fall into this category.

Not all providers, however, need to know such information. Their own rigorous and objective consideration of this question is crucial. For example, in the context of general program operation, even in a residential setting, providers do not need to know the HIV antibody status of any particular individual. General infection control procedures are adequate to ensure that HIV is not transmitted between participants or staff and will help protect people with HIV disease from casually transmitted infections that might pose a danger to their health. (See also Appendix C: *Infection Control.*)

The tools and lessons of a 12-step program are relevant to a wide range of personal issues. Strategies for dealing with fear work for all kinds of fear. Approaches addressing obsession work for all kinds of obsession. Confrontations of denial will work for all kinds of denial. It is entirely possible for providers to share experience, strength, and hope that is meaningful and helpful to HIV-infected people, without actually knowing if participants have HIV disease. Sharing in a general way may be adequate and appropriate.

When a provider is involved in the medical care of participants—completing physical assessments and examinations, making medical diagnoses, and offering treatment recommendations—knowing an individual's HIV antibody status will be necessary. Providers involved in intensive, long-term, helping relationships, such as individual psychotherapy, are also likely to find this information relevant for success in their work. In other kinds of supportive relationships, such as social model recovery, group programs, community-based outreach, or brief psychotherapy, it may not be necessary for providers to know the antibody status of participants.

Providers who are informed about HIV disease, willing to listen to participants' concerns, and sympathetic and understanding about these issues can help participants learn to take responsibility for their lives. By the same token, however, providers must be willing to give over responsibility to participants when they are able to take it for themselves. Allowing participants to choose whether to share HIV-related personal information can be healing and empowering even if the decision is to hold the information privately. (See also Chapter 8: *Looking at Policy.*)

Providing Ongoing Support

Some individuals in recovery who go through the process of HIV antibody testing will do so without great distress or discomfort. The relief of "finally knowing" may be considerable. Many of those who receive antibody negative test results will be able to lay to rest fears or concerns about past behaviors, and make new and healthier commitments for the future. These individuals will need little follow-up or ongoing attention concerning HIV-related issues.

Others, however, may test negative while they are in the six month window period of infection. Rather than settling their concerns, they may find themselves preparing for a long period of anxiety, as they wait out the window period before taking a second test.

Still others who test antibody negative will experience "survivor guilt." This painful and confusing response is not uncommon in people who have watched many friends become ill or die, but who themselves have remained uninfected despite their past participation in risky behaviors. Individuals struggling with a sense of guilt, disappointment, or abandonment after testing negative often face profound spiritual challenges and benefit from ongoing support and understanding.

For people in recovery who test antibody positive, a lifelong adjustment is required. Can they hold on to serenity and recovery when diagnosed with another life-threatening disease? If they are rejected by friends, family or members of the recovery program, will their sobriety remain intact? As new challenges arise, will their programs of recovery offer support?

The antibody test may be seen as the first step in the process of acknowledging the true threat of HIV disease. It is also one of the most delicate steps, and if handled improperly, can threaten not only recovery, but emotional health, spiritual strength, and life itself. Recovery providers can ensure that throughout the testing process—from making a decision about whether to test to living with test results—participants understand their options, take appropriate actions to implement the options they choose, and protect their sobriety.

Talking about Antibody Testing

Participants will ask questions about antibody testing, and providers should consider the discussions that follow an opportunity to share information about testing. This section includes questions providers can ask to learn about participants' concerns. These questions are not designed to be comprehensive or to provide an explicit "recipe" for responding to participants. Rather, they represent a series of suggestions that can be useful in discussions about HIV antibody testing. Not all questions will be relevant or necessary in every situation.

Thinking about Taking the Test

It is essential at this time to carefully assess participants' decision-making abilities. To do this, providers need to offer background information about antibody testing, support participants in whatever decisions they make, help participants apply "rigorous honesty" to HIV-related issues, and maintain a focus on recovery and sobriety.

Gathering information from participants

- What do you know about the antibody test?
- What information will the test give you?
- What are the limitations of the test? What information will it not give you?

Risk reduction education

- Do you understand what the risk behaviors for HIV are? Can you describe them to me?
- Can you tell me about your own HIV risk behaviors? What behaviors are you concerned about?
- Are you continuing to engage in any of these behaviors? Do you know how to protect yourself from HIV disease?

Assessing potential problems

- If you do decide to take the test, how will that feel?
- If you decide not to be tested, how will that feel?
- To whom can you talk about these concerns?
- What will happen if you test positive? What if you test negative?
- Do you have concerns about the process of taking the test, waiting for results, or receiving results?

- Is thinking about the antibody test affecting your recovery or sobriety in any way?
- Is this the best time for you to take the test? What are some reasons for taking it now or for waiting?

Follow-up

- If you want to talk about these concerns further, I hope you'll feel free to talk to me.
- Do you want any help finding an HIV counselor to talk to?

Making the Decision to Be Tested

During this period, assist participants in understanding the HIV antibody testing process and in planning both the testing itself and the support they may need during this process. Help participants identify healthy coping strategies they have used and can use in times of stress. Keep a steady focus on sobriety and recovery.

Practical issues

- Do you know the difference between anonymous and confidential testing? Which will be better for you?
- Where can you go to take the test? Do you know how to set up an appointment?

Planning and preparation

- Who will you talk to about your decision to be tested? Is there anyone you don't want to share this with?
- How will you feel while you are waiting for the test results? What can you do to support yourself during that time?
- What ways of coping have you used in the past when faced with difficulties? Which of these have been healthy?
- Have you had episodes of relapse in sobriety before? If so, what were the circumstances of the relapse? Were these similar to what you might experience in seeking the antibody test?
- What will you need to do during the antibody testing process to check on your recovery and sobriety?
- What will happen if you test antibody positive?

Action steps to cope with the process

- Let's identify people you can talk to about being tested, including at least one person knowledgeable about the Twelve Steps.
- You might want to write out a list of some of the ways you can support yourself during the testing process, and refer back to the list when you need support.
- I would like to talk to you at least a couple of times during the waiting period. Can we set up a time to do that now?

Waiting for Results

This may be a difficult, potentially slippery time for participants. Are they taking the necessary steps to protect sobriety? For example, talking to trusted friends during the waiting period and immediately after disclosure will be very important, and isolation during these times could make a difficult situation worse.

Providing support

- Do you want to talk about how things are going now that you're waiting for your test results?

Coping strategies

- During the waiting period, what coping strategies are working?
- Are you having any new difficulties with eating or sleeping? Are you feeling upset or depressed?
- Do you need to identify other ways of coping, or are things going well?

Sobriety

- Has taking the HIV antibody test affected your feelings or thoughts about sobriety and recovery?
- Are you thinking about drinking more in this period than you were before you took the test?

Planning and preparation

- When is your appointment to get your test results? Do you need to make any special preparations for that time?

- When you get your results, be sure to get additional written information from the counselor. The counselor may have pamphlets or books that explain more about your test results, or telephone numbers you can call for further support or information.

After Receiving Results

In the post-test counseling session, people often don't "get" all of the information provided. For the person who tests negative, this can happen because the relief is so profound. For the person who tests positive, even when this is the expected result, the shock can be surprisingly powerful. After the test, providers should help participants understand their results, deal with their emotional response, and plan for the future.

Checking in

- How are you feeling now that you've received your test result?
- Have you been able to talk about your results with a trusted friend or a counselor? Would you like to discuss any of this with me?

After testing antibody negative

- How are you feeling about your negative test result? Do you understand what it means?
- Do you know whether you might be in the window period of infection?
- Are you clear about how to protect yourself from HIV infection in the future?
- Some people who test antibody negative find themselves feeling sad, depressed, or anxious. Have you had any reactions like this?
- How are you feeling about your sobriety and recovery?
- Are you thinking about drinking more now than you were before you took the test?

After testing antibody positive

- It is important for you to see a physician and have your health evaluated. Do you know who to see and how to set up an appointment? May I give you referrals for medical care?

- Can you afford medical care? May I give you referrals for low-cost medical care?
- It may seem difficult to deal with a doctor now. Can we start by setting out a plan to help you deal with HIV disease?
- Would you like a referral to an agency that can provide individual or group support specifically for people with HIV disease?

The small steps providers can take—being willing to address the issues, to listen, to ask and answer questions, and to let participants make their own choices about coping with HIV disease—can contribute immensely to the well being of the general recovery community as well as to the lives of individual participants.

APPENDIX C

INFECTION CONTROL

In most states, licensing standards and legal obligations require service agencies and residential programs to prevent the transmission of all blood-borne diseases—including HIV infection and various types of hepatitis—as well as the transmission of airborne or other diseases. While HIV disease focuses attention on these issues, it has not, in fact, raised new obligations. The following guidelines should already be in place in recovery programs. One of the opportunities presented by the HIV epidemic is that of evaluating current infection control standards to ensure that they are adequate and comply with laws and licensing regulations.

As stated in Chapter 4: *Facts about HIV Disease,* HIV is not casually transmitted. People become infected with HIV only when they take into their bodies the blood, semen, or vaginal secretions of an HIV-infected person. Such contact rarely happens except when people have sexual intercourse or share needles during injection drug use. In a residential or agency setting, there is also a small risk that people may have contact with blood in first aid situations.

The guidelines included in this chapter will also help people with HIV disease stay healthy. Bacteria, fungi, and viruses that might not be a problem to a healthy person can make an HIV-infected person seriously ill. A good infection control plan represents an important commitment to health and well-being throughout a program.

Routine Daily Contact

Since HIV is not casually transmitted, special precautions are generally not necessary during normal daily contact.

Spills of Blood or Body Fluids

Any time there has been a spill of blood or "bloody body fluids" (in which visible blood is present), special care should be taken. Avoid having direct skin contact with blood or bloody body fluids: wear latex gloves to clean up such spills if possible.

Spills can be cleaned with a 1:10 solution of household bleach. This would be 1 part bleach (such as Clorox or Purex) to 9 parts water. (Each "part" is an equal amount of liquid.) Paper towels or other disposable cloths should be used for cleaning.

Wash hands after any contact with blood or bloody body fluids, using regular hand soap and warm water.

First Aid

When providing first aid, avoid direct contact with blood or bloody body fluids. Latex gloves should be made available for first aid procedures that involve contact with another person's blood.

Cuts and abrasions on the skin, particularly on the hands, should be covered with bandages when possible. If bandaging is not possible, avoid any direct contact with blood or bloody body fluids in the area of the cut or abrasion.

When possible, disposable thermometers or thermometer sleeves should be used. These are usually available at pharmacies. If disposable thermometers are not available, usual methods of disinfection are adequate. To disinfect a thermometer, rinse it in warm, soapy water, then rinse it in plain water, and then soak it in isopropyl alcohol for 20 minutes or more.

CPR and Mouth-to-Mouth Resuscitation

There are no cases of HIV transmission through CPR or mouth-to-mouth resuscitation. However, there is a slight chance that there could be an exchange of blood during mouth-to-mouth resuscitation. This might happen if the injured person is bleeding internally or is bleeding in or around the mouth, and if the person doing the resuscitation also has an open sore or cut in the mouth area.

While there are no reported cases of HIV transmission through CPR, there are other diseases which could be spread in this manner. Therefore, people who might perform CPR in the normal course of their employment should be provided with special masks with one-way valves and training on how to use these masks. The masks will prevent the slight risk of HIV transmission, as well as the transmission of other diseases, during mouth-to-mouth resuscitation.

When a mask is not be available, rescuers are reminded that the actual risk of HIV transmission is quite small during mouth-to-mouth resuscitation, even if the patient does have HIV infection. In such situations, rescuers must make the most ethical choice they can about whether to respond. Some professionals, such as first responders—paramedics, police officers, firefighters, and lifeguards—may have a duty to respond in these situations.

Food Preparation

People with HIV disease can prepare foods and eat without posing a risk to others. Unless there is an accident involving a bleeding wound, no special precautions are necessary.

It is a good idea for anyone preparing meals to wash his or her hands before handling food and to avoid tasting food with fingers or cooking spoons. HIV will not be transmitted in these ways, but other diseases, such as colds and flu, can be.

Bathroom Use

People with HIV disease can safely share bathrooms with others. Body wastes should be flushed promptly. Used menstrual products should be wrapped in tissue or toilet paper and placed in the trash. Paper towels should be available for drying hands after washing. Once again, any incidents involving bleeding should be handled appropriately, and any blood spills should be cleaned promptly.

Housekeeping

General cleaning

General cleaning should be done on a regular basis, at least weekly. Keep floors swept, carpets and rugs vacuumed, and surfaces, including moldings, dusted. Dust, dirt, and pet hair can cause breathing difficulties for people with lung disease.

Kitchen

Counters should be cleaned regularly with scouring powder or another cleaning agent. Sponges or cloths used in the kitchen should not be used in the bathroom. Dirty or stained sponges or cloths should be discarded and replaced.

Floors should be mopped weekly. Spills should be cleaned promptly. Paper towels can be used for cleaning smaller spills on floors. Sponges used on countertops should not be used on floors.

The insides of refrigerators should be cleaned with soap and water to control molds, which might be dangerous to someone with HIV infection.

Paper towels should be available for drying hands after washing. As people attend more to ecological issues, there is a tendency to use cloth towels in the kitchen. In residential programs, this is not recommended. Kitchen waste baskets should be emptied regularly, at least every other day.

No special measures are needed for washing dishes. Washing in hot, soapy water will keep them clean and help protect people with HIV disease from illnesses carried by other people. Dishes can be air dried in a dish drainer, or heat dried in a dishwasher. Do not use cloth towels for dish-drying.

Bathroom

Floors should be mopped weekly. To kill athlete's foot fungus, bath and shower floors should be disinfected weekly with a 1:10 solution of bleach.

Waste baskets should be emptied regularly, at least every other day. Baskets should not be allowed to overflow so that trash is spilling onto the floor.

Personal Hygiene

Residents should not share towels or washcloths, toothbrushes, or razors. Linens should be laundered between users. Towels and washcloths should be laundered at least weekly.

Pets

People with HIV disease may become ill cleaning cat litter boxes, tropical fish tanks, or bird cages. It is best for someone else to clean up after pets. Cats or other pets should never be allowed to walk on kitchen tables or counters.

Health Care Workers

Health care workers who draw blood, give shots, or perform other invasive procedures should be completely familiar with infection control guidelines for their professions. These guidelines, when carefully followed, will prevent most cases of occupational exposure to HIV.[1]

References

1. For a thorough description of infection control guidelines for health care workers, see: Centers for Disease Control. Update: universal precautions for prevention of transmission of human immunodeficiency virus, hepatitis B virus, and other blood-borne pathogens in health care settings. *Morbidity and Mortality Weekly Report.* 37 (1988): 337-382, 387-388.

APPENDIX D

PARTICIPANT TRAINING TOOLS

This appendix includes outlines for four training sessions, each reviewing an HIV-related issue that may affect people in recovery. By following the instructions in the session outline, providers will be able to guide participants through a learning experience.

The first two sessions are good general activities for most groups. *Session #1 – What is Safer Sex?* reviews facts about HIV prevention and safer sex. *Session #2 – Safer Sex: Condoms and Barriers* provides more detailed information about condom and barrier use in HIV prevention, and gives participants a chance to "practice" using condoms and barriers in a non-sexual setting. Recovery programs are encouraged to provide thorough HIV education to all participants, and these sessions can help in that effort.

Talking about sex with participants in recovery can be difficult. People do not want to admit to past experiences they find embarrassing or shameful, or that they may lack sexual experience. The explicit discussions necessary in HIV education make some people uncomfortable: talking about sexual issues in an open, direct way within a group of people, especially a mixed group of men and women, will be so unusual for some people that it will cause them considerable anxiety. In response to these conflicts, participants may withdraw, act out, or express judgmental or negative attitudes about others. Racist, sexist, or homophobic remarks are not uncommon in discussions about sex and HIV disease with people in recovery. (See also Chapter 5: *Talking about Sexuality.*)

The trainings included here emphasize early recovery. However, with minor adjustments, the sessions can be adapted for individuals with longer term recovery and in group outpatient or day treatment mental health settings, in drug treatment communities, or for clients of community-based organizations.

Each facilitator will find his or her own way of dealing with these challenges. Remember that one of the potential benefits of sex education in recovery is the modelling of socially appropriate behavior. It will be helpful for participants to understand that they can talk about sexuality in a forthright manner that is respectful to themselves, to their brothers and sisters in recovery, and to other people.

Sessions #3 and #4 of this section are for more specialized situations. *Session #3 – Deciding about the HIV Antibody Test* addresses how people in recovery can make informed decisions about whether or not to take the HIV antibody test. It will be most useful in a group setting in which individuals have already had some discussions about the antibody test. *Session #4 – Responding to HIV-Related Loss and Grief* will be most useful in situations where someone who participants know well has died or become seriously ill because of HIV-related illnesses.

In many recovery settings, staff turnover is frequent, and participants are present only for short periods of time. In these situations, it will be most useful to cover the basics about HIV transmission and prevention as an introduction to every session. In addition, it is helpful to make available handouts describing safer sex activities, and instructions for needle cleaning, and for condom and latex dam use, for anyone who has not seen these handouts before. (See the pages following 215 for these training session materials.)

These sessions emphasize *active learning.* Most people learn more easily when they are actively involved in their learning through discussion, interaction with each other, and hands-on practice.

The following suggestions will be useful for providers planning to carry out one or more of the sessions:

- Start by reading session instructions all the way through. Then evaluate whether this session is "right" for your participant group. If not, feel free to adapt the session so that it fits better, or to find another way to teach the material.
- Be sure to have your demonstration, and handouts and pamphlets prepared ahead of time.
- As you go through the sessions, try not to read from the outline. People will be able to listen better if you can talk to them in a

normal, conversational way. A lot of information has been included here to give you background on an issue. You do not necessarily need to cover every point written in the outline.

- If it seems necessary, cover the basics about HIV transmission and prevention before every session.

Three additional guidelines will be relevant for all of these sessions and will assure that trainings are effective.

KEEP IT SIMPLE. Speak in simple terms. Present new ideas and concepts simply. Don't rush, and don't put too much information into the session. It is better to simplify a session and give people less information that they will be able to learn well, then to rush a session and fill it with more information than people can handle.

NO JUDGMENTS. Participants are often asked to share personal opinions and experiences in these sessions. If they feel a trainer is being judgmental, they will be less involved in the session. Be sure to listen to what people say with an open mind and heart.

LET PARTICIPANTS TEACH THEMSELVES. The session will be more effective if the group can learn from the activities and ideas they share. As the group "leader," you are there to serve the group in its effort to learn new information. Be careful not to take over or dictate to the group.

SESSION #1 – WHAT IS SAFER SEX?

OVERVIEW

TIME. 60 minutes.

PURPOSE. To help participants understand what safer sex is.

TRAINEE KNOWLEDGE. No previous knowledge needed.

MATERIALS. Collect the following materials for use during this session:

- Butcher paper.
- Different colored markers.
- Masking tape.
- Lots of pieces of plain paper about 8 inches x 3 inches, or 5 inch x 7 inch index cards. You can cut plain typing paper into strips of three pieces and your paper will be the right size. It's okay if the sheets of paper are a little different in size. They can also be different colors.
- Handouts: "Using Condoms," "More about Using Condoms," "Using Latex Barriers," "Cleaning Needles and Works," and "Safe and Unsafe Sexual Activities." (These handouts—which may be photocopied for the session—are included after page 215.)

PREPARATION. You may want to make the "Safe Sex Scale," mentioned on page 190, ahead of time.

SUGGESTIONS FOR THIS SESSION. This is a good basic session for any group. It reviews what safer sex is and why it is important. This session, as written, requires at least eight people to participate. If your group is smaller, you will need to make some adaptations.

1. GETTING STARTED

A. REVIEW YOUR PROGRAM'S GUIDELINES ABOUT SEXUAL ACTIVITY.

Most programs suggest participants avoid new sexual relationships in early sobriety. Most have rules against sexual activities between participants.

B. Explain what the group will be doing today.

The group will be talking about safer sex. Let the group know that no assumptions are being made about whether participants are currently sexually active or not. This is important information for anyone who is or may some day be sexually active.

2. HIV Basics

A. Defining HIV and AIDS.

HIV is the virus that causes AIDS. The virus attacks the immune system. People with HIV disease and AIDS can develop illnesses that do not affect individuals with healthy immune systems. A person with HIV disease often looks and feels perfectly healthy many years after infection. Over that time, the virus acts slowly, gradually weakening the immune system, and mild to moderate symptoms may develop. AIDS is usually diagnosed at an advanced stage of infection, when the immune system is badly damaged and serious illness is likely.

B. How HIV is passed from person to person.

First, through unprotected sexual intercourse—vaginal, oral, or anal—that involves an exchange of blood, semen, or vaginal secretions. "Unprotected" means without a condom or latex barrier. Second, through sharing needles or equipment during injection drug use, or through other exchanges of blood or bloody body fluids. Finally, a pregnant woman with HIV disease can pass the virus on to her fetus during pregnancy, or her child may be infected during the birth process.

C. How to prevent HIV transmission.

Do not have unprotected intercourse. Use condoms or latex barriers for all acts of intercourse—vaginal, anal, and oral.

Do not share needles or equipment during injection drug use. If sharing is absolutely necessary, clean needles with bleach before sharing.

3. What Is Safer Sex?

A. Ask the group: "What is safer sex? What is it for?"

Try to get several different answers from participants. You can give some answers of your own if the group is quiet. Be patient and give participants a minute to think about the question. Possible answers include:

- Sex that does not involve a risk of getting sexually transmitted diseases (STDs).
- Sex that protects you from HIV infection.
- Sex using condoms or latex barriers.
- Sexual activities like fantasy, massage, and masturbation.

4. Why Is This Important?

A. Ask the group: "Why is it important for people to know about safer sex?"

Try to get several different answers from participants. You can give some of your own if the group does not come up with answers. Possible answers include:

- So people can choose to protect themselves from AIDS or other STDs.
- Because some STDs can be very dangerous.
- Because it is important for people to know about healthy sex and to be able to talk about it.
- To save lives.

5. Reasons People Have Sex

A. Ask the group: "Why do people have sex?"

Try to get several different answers from participants. You can give some of your own if the group does not come up with answers. Possible answers include:

- To feel good physically.
- To feel good emotionally.
- To be close to someone.

- To relax.
- Because it is expected.

B. Ask the group: "Are there other things people can do, besides sex, that will fulfill these wishes or desires?"

Try to get several different answers from participants. You can give some of your own if the group does not come up with answers. Possible answers include:

- Find other ways of being close to people—talk honestly with someone, take a quiet walk with someone, attend an AA meeting.
- Find other ways of feeling good physically—exercise, rest, meditate.
- Find other ways of feeling good emotionally—practice a program of recovery, work on building self-esteem.

C. Remember:

Sexuality is a wonderful aspect of life. The goal of this exercise is not to substitute non-sexual activities for sexual ones. Rather, the goal is to understand that each of us has many choices about how to respond to different desires, and sex is only one of these responses.

6. Listing Sexual Activities

A. Break into small groups.

Break the large group into smaller groups of four to six people each. You need two or more small groups for this activity. If you have a mixed group of men and women, the facilitator can choose to mix the small groups or keep them separated by gender.

B. Give a different colored marker to each group, and a bunch of paper strips.

The goal is to create groups with different identities. The easiest way of doing this is to ensure that different groups have different paper colors: a red group, a blue group, a green group.

C. Ask the groups to come up with a long list of sexual and sensual activities.

There are many different activities that people enjoy that are related to sexual and sensual feelings. One of the ways to understand more about safer sex is to think more openly about what activities can be considered sexual or sensual. Group members should work together to decide what these activities are and to write each separate activity on a separate piece of paper.

D. Encourage a little competition.

Encourage the groups to compete with each other to come up with the most activities or the most creative ideas.

7. "The Safer Sex Scale"

A. Post the "Scale" on the wall.

While people are working in their small groups, tape the "Safer Sex Scale" up on the wall. To make the scale, cut a long piece of paper—about 10 feet long—from a roll of paper, or post together several pieces of butcher paper. Mark on the paper, going from left to right, the numbers 1 to 10. By the number "1," write "Completely Safe." By the number "10," write "Completely Unsafe."

B. Finish the small group activity begun above.

When the small groups have finished their lists, or after five to 10 minutes, ask them to bring their attention to the full group.

C. Explain the "Safer Sex Scale."

The scale ranges from 1 to 10, where 1 represents completely safe activities and 10 represents completely unsafe activities. The numbers in between 1 and 10 measure "relative" risk, so an activity that is rated 8 is more risky than one rated 4.

D. Have groups post their activities up on the scale.

Each group should tape their activities up on the scale under the number that best describes the risk level of the activity. Every-one in the small group must agree on where to place each activity. If group members can't reach agreement, they should set the activity aside. However, it is all right for one group to disagree with another group.

Typically when this activity is done, there is a lot of agreement about where certain activities belong on the scale. There will be a long list under 1 and a long list under 10. There will be more confusion and argument about everything in between.

8. Discussion

A. Ask the group: "What have you learned from this activity?"

If participants are slow to respond, you might suggest some of the following answers:

- There are a lot more sexual or sensual activities than we thought there were.
- No one can agree on what safer sex is.
- There is lots of agreement about some activities.
- If someone says they practice safer sex, you don't necessarily know what they're talking about.
- Risk may vary depending on an individual's role in an activity. For example, "receptive anal intercourse without a condom" is more risky than "active anal intercourse with a condom," even though both activities have HIV-related risks.
- Very specific descriptions may be necessary to evaluate risk. For example, "anal intercourse" is less descriptive than "receptive anal intercourse without a condom."

B. Ask the group: "About which activities was there disagreement in the small groups?"

Discuss why these activities were harder to place on the scale. Clarify misinformation as necessary.

C. Ask the group: "What disagreements are there between the small groups?"

Let people from the different groups discuss their differences. When people talk about these differences, is it easier to understand why two groups may have ranked similar activities differently?

D. Ask the group: "Does this activity tell us anything about the differences between people and the risks they take in their lives?"

Try to get several different answers from participants. You can give some of your own if the group does not come up with answers.

Possible answers include:

- What seems very risky to one person might seem fairly safe to another.
- There are no absolute answers about some activities. People cope differently with unclear information.

9. Handouts

A. Distribute handouts to participants.

Go over the handouts briefly, and clarify them in response to questions from participants.

10. Closure

A. Acknowledge that this kind of discussion can be difficult for people.

Participants may have thoughts or feelings about the topics of this training later. They may have questions that were not answered in the session. Encourage participants to talk to one another, or to counselors, to help reason these things out. Be available yourself to talk with people if they wish, or provide the name of someone else who can do so.

B. Support people in taking care of themselves in many different ways.

Knowing about safer sex, including how to use condoms is a way to take care of ourselves, like knowing about exercise and nutrition.

C. Remind people that maintaining sobriety is the foundation upon which they are building their lives.

Review program guidelines about sexuality and intimacy, and encourage people to protect their sobriety above all else.

SESSION #2 – SAFER SEX: CONDOMS AND BARRIERS

OVERVIEW

TIME. 60 minutes

PURPOSE. To teach participants about condoms and latex barriers, and how they are used.

TRAINEE KNOWLEDGE. It is best if participants have already had a session on safer sex (such as Session #1 of this series). If they already know what safer sex is and why it is important, more time can be spent on practice with condoms and latex barriers.

MATERIALS. Collect the following materials for use during this session:

- Condoms (two for each participant).
- Latex barriers (one for each participant), *and/or*
- Non-lubricated condoms to "cut down." (See page 218 for explanation.)
- Tissue or paper towels to wipe hands if lubricated condoms are used.
- *Optional, but a good idea:* Samples of water-based lubricants.
- *Optional:* Several dildos, bananas, or cucumbers.
- Handouts: "Using Condoms," "More about Using Condoms," "Using Latex Barriers," "Cleaning Needles and Works," and "Safe and Unsafe Sexual Activities." (These handouts—which may be photocopied for the session—are included after page 215.)

PREPARATION. It is essential that the facilitator know how to properly demonstrate condom use. For assistance with this, check with local STD clinics, Planned Parenthood clinics, or other health providers who can help facilitators learn to present this information properly. Before the session, practice with these materials to become comfortable demonstrating their use.

SUGGESTIONS FOR THIS SESSION. During the session, it's okay for people to laugh, be embarrassed, or have fun. Allow participants these or other emotional responses while maintaining the focus on proper use of condoms and latex barriers.

1. Getting Started

A. Review your program's guidelines about sexual activity.

Most programs suggest participants avoid new sexual relationships in early sobriety. Most have rules against sexual activities between participants.

B. Explain what the group will be doing today.

The group will be talking about safer sex, condoms, and latex barriers. Let the group know that no assumptions are being made about whether participants are currently sexually active or not. This is important information for anyone who is or may some day be sexually active.

2. HIV Basics

A. Defining HIV and AIDS.

HIV is the virus that causes AIDS. The virus attacks the immune system. People with HIV disease and AIDS can develop illnesses that do not affect individuals with healthy immune systems. A person with HIV disease often looks and feels perfectly healthy many years after infection. Over that time, the virus acts slowly, gradually weakening the immune system, and mild to moderate symptoms may develop. AIDS is usually diagnosed at an advanced stage of infection, when the immune system is badly damaged and serious illness is likely.

B. How HIV is passed from person to person.

First, through unprotected sexual intercourse—vaginal, oral, or anal—that involves an exchange of blood, semen, or vaginal secretions. "Unprotected" means without a condom or latex barrier. Second, through sharing needles or equipment during injection drug use, or through other exchanges of blood or bloody body fluids. Finally, a pregnant woman with HIV disease can pass the virus on to her fetus during pregnancy, or her child may be infected during the birth process.

C. How to prevent HIV transmission.

Do not have unprotected intercourse. Use condoms or latex barriers for all acts of intercourse—vaginal, anal, and oral.

Do not share needles or equipment during injection drug use. If sharing is absolutely necessary, clean needles with bleach before sharing.

3. What Is Safer Sex?

A. Ask the group: "What is safer sex? What is it for?"

Try to get several different answers from participants. You can give some answers of your own if the group is quiet. Be patient and give participants a minute to think about the question. Possible answers include:

- Sex that does not involve a risk of getting sexually transmitted diseases (STDs).
- Sex that protects you from HIV infection.
- Sex using condoms or latex barriers.
- Sexual activities like fantasy, massage, and masturbation.

B. Hand out "Safe and Unsafe Sexual Activities." Answer any questions people may have about what is and is not safe.

If participants have not already had a session on safer sex, you will need to spend more time going over this list.

4. Why Is This Important?

A. Ask the group: "Why is it important for people to know about safer sex?"

Try to get several different answers from participants. You can give some of your own if the group does not come up with answers. Possible answers include:

- So people can choose to protect themselves from AIDS or other STDs.

- Because some STDs can be very dangerous.
- Because it is important for people to know about healthy sex and to be able to talk about it.
- To save lives.

5. Let's Practice: Condom Use

A. Demonstrate how to use a condom.

It is essential that the person doing the demonstration knows how to demonstrate proper condom use and feels comfortable doing so.

Use a model penis, such as a dildo, for the demonstration. Or use the index and middle fingers of one hand, a banana, or a cucumber as a "substitute penis." Be sure to tell people the banana or the fingers are substituting for a penis!

Remind participants that condoms should be used only one time and then discarded.

B. Demonstrate how to use water-based lubricant.

Place a small amount of lubricant inside the tip of the condom to increase sensation on the penis. Apply a moderate amount on the lower two-thirds of the outside of the condom. If a condom is over-lubricated, or is lubricated right up to the point near the man's body, it may slip off.

It is important for people to *see* what the bottle or jar of lubricant looks like. A good lubricant to use is *K-Y Jelly,* easily available at most drug stores. Other popular water-based lubricants are *Probe* and *Astro-Glide.*

C. Describe nonoxynol-9.

For many years, HIV educators have recommended using lubricants containing nonoxynol-9 spermicide. This spermicide, which kills HIV, is used as "insurance" in case the condom breaks. Recently, there have been many reports of allergies to nonoxynol-9 and people developing rashes in response. If a man develops a rash on his penis, a woman develops a rash in her vagina, or men or women develop rashes in the anus as a result of using nonoxynol-9, the risk of HIV transmission will actually *increase*. The virus could enter through the tiny cuts or sores of the rash.

People can test lubricants with nonoxynol-9 to be sure they do not cause a rash. Simply put a little of the lubricant on the inside of the arm, and check it again in 24 hours. If a rash has developed, do not use that lubricant.

D. Small group practice.

Break the group into small groups of three, and give everyone a condom. Ask them to demonstrate how to use the condom to the other participants in their group. Everyone should practice once.

Encourage people to notice the sensation of the condom on their fingers. Tell them to close their eyes and touch their condom-covered fingers, and to note the sensation they feel. If you have lubricant to pass around, ask participants to compare the feeling of the condom with and without lubricant.

E. Full group discussion.

As the groups finish, draw their attention back to the full group. People can stay in their small groups. Remind people that condoms should be used for vaginal or anal intercourse, and also for oral intercourse performed on a man. Non-lubricated condoms are preferred for oral sex because the lubricants taste terrible.

Answer any questions. Hand out paper towels to dry hands if lubricated condoms were used.

6. Let's Practice: Latex Barriers

A. Describe latex barriers.

Explain that latex "barriers" are used for oral sex on a woman, or oral-anal sex on anybody. Basically, the barrier keeps vaginal secretions, blood, or germs from being passed from one partner to another.

In mouth-to-vagina sex, HIV and other STDs can be passed from one person to another in vaginal secretions or blood. The latex barrier can keep these fluids from being passed between people.

In oral-anal sex, it is easy for certain diseases to be passed, especially parasites. Latex barriers are believed to prevent the passing of parasites or other diseases during oral-anal sex.

B. Describe the barriers that are available: dental dams, "cut-down" condoms, and plastic wrap.

Some people use latex dental dams for safer sex. These are available through dental supply houses and some stores that sell sexual products. However, the dental dams are not as thin or shear as latex condoms, and they have not been tested as latex condoms have been to ensure that they prevent the transmission of HIV and other germs.

It is important to note that there is no scientific proof that dental dams prevent HIV. It is reasonable to assume, however, that if the barrier keeps fluids from passing between people, it will keep a virus like HIV, which lives in fluids, from passing between people.

A better choice for a latex dam is a "cut-down" condom. Condoms are thinner than dental dams and have shown in studies to be effective in stopping HIV transmission. To modify a condom, simply take a non-lubricated condom, cut it along one side, and unroll it to flatten it out.

Some people suggest using clear plastic wrap as a flat barrier. Plastic wrap, however, is easily torn or punctured, is permeable, and has never been tested as a disease-preventing material. A cut-down condom seems like a better choice.

C. Demonstrate how to use latex barrier.

You can use the palm of your hand to demonstrate use of the dam. Lay the barrier on your hand and massage your palm lightly with the fingers of your other hand. Tell participants that the palm of your hand is a substitute for a vulva or anus, and your fingers are a substitute for a tongue.

Remind participants that it is important to keep one side of the dam towards the partner and the other side towards themselves, and to avoid mixing up the sides. Some people make a small mark on one side of the barrier with a pen to remind them which side is which.

Latex barriers should be used only one time and then discarded.

D. Small group practice.

In small groups of three, have each person demonstrate how to use the latex or barrier. Again, encourage participants to close their eyes and notice the sensations as they touch the palms of their hands.

7. Discussion

A. Initial responses.

Ask how people feel about handling and talking about condoms and latex barriers. Encourage open and honest responses. Listen without judgment.

B. Ask the group: "What might keep people from using condoms or latex barriers?"

Encourage open and honest responses. Try to get several different answers from participants. You can offer some of your own if the group does not come up with answers. Possible answers include:

- Discomfort using them.
- Discomfort talking about using them.
- Doesn't seem that important.
- Denial about the risks of HIV infection or other STDs.

C. Ask the group: "Are there special issues for people new in sobriety that affect their ability to follow through in practicing safer sex and using condoms?"

Encourage open and honest responses. Try to get several different answers from participants. You can offer some of your own if the group does not come up with answers. Possible answers include:

- No experience having sober sex.
- Limited social skills ("I feel like I'm 12 years old.").
- Lack of support among others for practicing safer sex.

8. Closure

A. Acknowledge that this kind of discussion can be difficult for people.

Participants may have thoughts or feelings about this session later. They may have questions that were not answered. Encourage participants to talk to one another or to counselors to help reason things out. Be available yourself to talk with people if they wish, or provide the name of someone who can be available.

B. Support people in taking care of themselves in many ways.

Knowing about how to use condoms and barriers, and using them, is a way to take care of ourselves. This is similar to knowing about exercise and nutrition.

C. Remind people that maintaining sobriety is the most important thing in their lives.

Review program guidelines about sexuality and intimacy, and encourage people to protect their sobriety above all else.

SESSION #3 – DECIDING ABOUT THE HIV ANTIBODY TEST

OVERVIEW

TIME. 60 minutes

PURPOSE. To help participants consider the pros and cons of taking the HIV antibody test.

TRAINEE KNOWLEDGE. It is best if participants have already had some background on HIV disease. This might include a session on safer sex (see "Session #1" of this series). It might also include a basic presentation on HIV infection: what HIV is, how it is passed from person to person, how it is prevented, and what the HIV antibody test measures.

MATERIALS. Collect the following materials for use during this session:

- Butcher paper.
- Markers.
- Masking tape.
- Or a blackboard and chalk.

PREPARATION. Read Appendix B: *HIV Antibody Testing* and the short essay, "HIV Antibody Testing in Early Recovery" (page 202). Prepare three sheets of butcher paper. Label one, "Going to take the test." Label the second, "Not going to take the test." Label the third, "Undecided."

SUGGESTIONS FOR THIS SESSION. This session is designed for participants in programs where the issue of HIV antibody testing has been raised. The main purpose of the session is to help people stop and think about antibody testing so they can make "informed decisions" about whether or not to take the antibody test. An informed decision is a decision that takes into account a variety of issues, including the pros and cons of taking the test for a person in recovery.

Other tests for HIV infection may become available. This exercise can be adapted to address "Finding Out if You Have HIV Infection," if antibody testing is not the test being used.

1. Getting Started

A. Before the session: Read to yourself the following short essay on HIV antibody testing and recovery.

HIV can be a frustrating issue for recovery providers. Sometimes it seems there is little one can do to help participants seeking reassurance, information, or advice.

The HIV antibody test feels like something concrete that providers can offer people. "Get the test. Find out if you've been infected. If you have, you can get treatments to help you."

But for the person new to recovery, the issues are more complex. Providers must consider what effect any new health concerns—including a positive HIV antibody test result—might have on newly sober individuals.

If a person learns he or she is infected with HIV, powerful feelings usually come up. Typical reactions include fear, anger, doubt, guilt, hopelessness, and despair. Thoughts of suicide are common, although these usually last only a short time. How well can the newly sober person deal with these intense emotions? Will he or she be able to maintain sobriety? Or will the information be too great a challenge to the fragile state of early recovery?

People in early recovery are already coping with a life-threatening illness. Alcoholism is a disease without a cure, but there is a successful treatment: regular participation in 12-step or other programs of recovery. In thinking about antibody testing, participants have to ask the question, "Will I be able to stay in treatment for alcoholism if I am also confronted with a second life-threatening illness, HIV infection, which has no known cure?" In some cases, it may be better for a person to wait until he or she is more stable in sobriety—perhaps after six months or more of continuous sobriety—before deciding whether or not to take the HIV antibody test.

It is true there are new treatments available for HIV infection, which slow the progression of the disease. There are also treatments for many of the specific conditions that commonly develop in people with HIV disease. None of these treatments cure HIV infection nor do they completely stop its progression. And they do not work equally well for everyone.

What must be balanced in the decision, then, are two different dangers. The first is the danger to a person's sobriety if he or she is given a positive HIV antibody result. The second is the danger to the individual's health if he or she is antibody positive and delays treatment for HIV infection or its associated illnesses.

The decision about whether to take the test belongs to the individual at risk, not to a counselor, sponsor, friend, or program. There are pros and cons to taking the test. Other factors, including whether the testing is anonymous or confidential, and whether it occurs during very early recovery or at a later time, are part of the decision-making process as well. The healthiest path for participants is to make their own informed decisions and to support others in doing the same.

B. Before the session: Prepare the visual materials for the session.

Post the three prepared pieces of butcher paper. One is labeled, "Going to take the test," another, "Not going to take the test," and the third, "Undecided."

2. HIV Basics

A. Defining HIV and AIDS.

HIV is the virus that causes AIDS. The virus attacks the immune system. People with HIV disease and AIDS can develop illnesses that do not affect individuals with healthy immune systems. A person with HIV disease often looks and feels perfectly healthy many years after infection. Over that time, the virus acts slowly, gradually weakening the immune system, and mild to moderate symptoms may develop. AIDS is usually diagnosed at an advanced stage of infection, when the immune system is badly damaged and serious illness is likely.

B. How HIV is passed from person to person.

First, through unprotected sexual intercourse—vaginal, oral, or anal—that involves an exchange of blood, semen, or vaginal secretions. "Unprotected" means without a condom or latex barrier. Second, through sharing needles or equipment during injection drug use, or through other exchanges of blood or bloody body fluids. Finally, a pregnant woman with HIV disease can pass the virus on to her fetus during pregnancy, or her child may be infected during the birth process.

C. How to prevent HIV transmission.

Do not have unprotected intercourse. Use condoms or latex barriers for all acts of intercourse—vaginal, anal, and oral.

Do not share needles or equipment during injection drug use. If sharing is absolutely necessary, clean needles with bleach before sharing.

3. HIV and Alcohol Connections

A. Review background information about HIV-related risks and alcohol use.

Remind people that HIV disease is a true danger and could directly affect them.

Many people with histories of alcoholism have reasons to think about their HIV-related risk history. They may have used substances other than alcohol and shared needles at one time. They may have had unprotected sex with someone else who had HIV-related risks. They may not remember everything they have done in their past, so they may not know what their risks are.

4. The HIV Antibody Test

A. Background information.

A blood test is available that can detect antibodies to HIV, the virus that causes HIV disease and AIDS. Antibodies are specialized proteins in the blood that help to fight infection. If the test shows that HIV-specific antibodies are present in the blood, it means the person has been infected with HIV.

If the test does not show antibodies to HIV in the blood, it means one of two things: the person is not infected with HIV; or the person is infected, but has not yet developed antibodies. After a person is first infected with HIV, it usually takes between two weeks and six months for HIV antibodies to show up in his or her blood. In rare cases, it could take longer than six months.

HIV antibodies seem to help fight the infection for a period of time. After several months or years, as HIV weakens the ability of antibodies and other parts of the immune system to respond, an HIV-infected person can become ill.

B. Raise the question of HIV antibody testing.

Because of the chance that a participant may have some HIV-related risks in his or her background, some people in recovery programs decide to take the HIV antibody test. While this might be something participants want to think about, it is important that they think carefully before taking the test.

A positive antibody test means that a person has antibodies to HIV and is HIV-infected. Common responses include powerful emotions such as fear, anger, sadness, frustration, doubt, guilt, hopelessness, or despair. Some people think about suicide after getting a positive test result.

People in early recovery need to think about the effects a positive or negative test result might have on sobriety. Only when they have thought carefully about this can they make informed decisions about whether or not to take the antibody test, and when it would be best to take it.

5. Describe Today's Activity

A. Tell the Group: "This activity will look at some of the pros and cons of the antibody test for people new in recovery."

6. Prepare for the Activity

A. Break into three groups.

Break participants into three groups numbered #1, #2, and #3.

B. Define the role of each group.

Each group will "speak for" an imaginary person in early recovery. The three groups will have a discussion about the HIV antibody test.

Group #1 speaks for a person who *is* going to take the test. Group #2 speaks for a person who *is not* going to take the test. Group #3 speaks for a person who *is undecided* about the test. Imagine that all three people have a genuine, clear HIV-related risk, and therefore have good reason to consider taking the test.

C. How the groups interact.

Groups #1 and #2 help group #3 decide whether or not to take the test. The groups are not necessarily disagreeing about the issue. Groups #1 and #2 are trying to assist group #3 in whatever way is most helpful. Group #3's task is to remain genuinely undecided as long as possible. Participants will have about 15 minutes for this discussion.

7. The activity

A. Begin the activity among the groups.

B. Write down some of the comments.

As the groups provide good arguments for or against taking the test, or reasons that the issue is confusing, write these down on the appropriate pieces of butcher paper.

C. Help out if needed.

During the activity, if a group is having trouble with arguments for or against testing, help out with some ideas. Help each group play its role well. It is important that people know you are asking them to pretend they have certain beliefs in order to make this activity work. They may or may not believe the things they say in the activity.

Help make this an interactive and lively exercise. You can encourage some controversy between Groups #1 and #2, or some exasperating indecisiveness from Group #3. Don't be afraid of building a little drama between the groups if it helps people get involved in the activity.

After about 10 minutes, or when the activity has slowed down, move on to a discussion of the activity.

8. Discuss the Activity

A. Ask the group: "How did you feel being in the group you were in? Was it easy or difficult to act as if you believed the things your group talked about?"

There are no right or wrong answers to these questions. Help provide an opportunity for participants to express their feelings openly, without judgment.

B. Ask the group: "Are there good reasons for a person with an HIV-related risk history to decide not to take the antibody test?"

Depending on the responses of the group, contribute ideas or suggestions that help keep a balanced perspective. For example, if a group expresses the opinion that no one in early recovery should seek an antibody test, point out the benefits of early testing and intervention for someone with HIV disease. If the group insists that everyone in recovery should be tested, mention the challenges testing might pose to some people who are newly sober.

C. Ask the group: "What will be most helpful for the person who is undecided about whether or not to take the test?"

Try to get several different answers from participants. You can give some answers of your own if the group is quiet. Be patient and give participants a minute to think about the question. Possible answers include:

- Knowing the tools of the program and how to use them.
- Self-acceptance and the acceptance of others; the person is fine where he or she is right now.
- Patience, and time to consider the matter more fully.
- The person may need more information about HIV infection and antibody testing.

D. Ask the group: "What are the most important issues for people new in recovery who are considering taking the antibody test?"

In this discussion, help people see the risks antibody testing might present to someone new in recovery. Some participants may do best if they conclude "not to decide"—just for today. Others may be more secure in their sobriety, the security of their support systems, and their understanding of what the antibody test will mean in their lives.

9. Closure

A. Acknowledge that making the decision to test is complicated. Offer the following recommendations:

- Encourage anyone thinking about taking the antibody test to think carefully and to be sure their decision is an informed one.
- Encourage people to support other participants in the decision-making process and to avoid trying to make decisions for anyone else.
- Be available to talk with people about HIV antibody testing or other HIV-related issues if they wish, or provide the name of someone else who can talk with them.

SESSION #4 – RESPONDING TO HIV-RELATED GRIEF AND LOSS

OVERVIEW

TIME. 60 minutes

PURPOSE. To help participants deal with feelings related to the HIV-related death or anticipated death of someone they know.

TRAINEE KNOWLEDGE. No previous knowledge is necessary. It would be best if participants knew basic information about HIV (what it is, how it is transmitted, and how it is not transmitted). This will help them focus on the issues of grief and loss, rather than on basic information questions.

MATERIALS. Collect the following materials for use during this session:

- Butcher paper.
- Markers.
- Masking tape.

SUGGESTIONS FOR THIS SESSION. This session is designed for use in programs where a participant, staff member, or another person is known to have HIV disease. It will be useful when participants have expressed concerns about this person's welfare or anxiety about his or her possible death, or in other ways have indicated that they are experiencing grief about the person's HIV disease.

The session may be most helpful when the participants are deeply affected by the circumstances, perhaps at a time when the individual is quite ill or has died. The session is written with this situation in mind.

With minor adaptation, however, it could also be used in the case of an HIV-infected person who is still feeling healthy, but is experiencing loss in relationship to sexual or personal identity, or anticipatory grief about the likelihood of future illness. Other participants are likely to have emotional responses of their own if this situation is publicly acknowledged, and the session can help them address these concerns.

1. Getting Started

A. Acknowledge common experiences.

Acknowledge the circumstances that led to the scheduling of this special session: that a program participant is ill, for example, that someone close to the program has died of HIV disease.

B. Set the tone for a safe environment.

Acknowledge people for the work they are doing in recovery. People are dealing with "new" feelings in sobriety. There are major challenges that arise in coping with these feelings. This session will strive to be a place where people are supported for having feelings.

C. Define "confidentiality," and obtain agreements to maintain confidentiality.

To keep this a safe experience, everyone should agree to hold what is said here in confidence. What's said in this room stays in this room.

2. Talking about Feelings

A. The myth of "bad" feelings.

Feelings or thoughts that are uncomfortable or are related to past drinking may seem to be "bad." In early recovery, it often seems like it would be better not to have these feelings at all. One of the things participants learn in recovery is how to have all kinds of feelings, without evaluating them as "good" or "bad," and without responding by drinking.

B. Brainstorm about feelings.

Ask people to name some of the uncomfortable feelings or thoughts they have now or have had in the past. These may be the feelings to which they used to respond by drinking. Write the feelings out on butcher paper. Possible feelings include: anger, sadness, fear, anxiety, uncertainty.

3. Experiences of Loss

A. We have all experienced loss.

Everyone has experienced many losses over his or her lifetime. People in new recovery share the recent loss of their "good friend" alcohol.

B. When we experience loss, we grieve.

People in new recovery experience grief because of the loss of alcohol in their lives. Everyone has experienced other kinds of grief as well. It is important to learn new ways to deal with grief, other than drinking. By applying the principles of a recovery program, participants can learn that intense feelings can be survived, and that people can tolerate almost anything by living one day at a time.

C. Other losses experienced in our lives.

Ask if anyone would like to mention briefly other losses experienced in his or her life. This might include losses as children or as adults.

Write some of these down on butcher paper. List them in a general way: for example, write "moving" when someone talks about his family's move from Arlington to Los Angeles. Possible losses include: moving, the death of a pet, parental separation or divorce, the break-up of a friendship, the break-up of a romantic relationship or marriage, personal illness or disability, or the death of a friend or family member. This section should stay fairly brief—about five minutes.

4. What Is it Like to Grieve?

A. Acknowledge the experiences people have shared.

Comment on the experiences of the group—for example, whether there are many different types of loss, whether these are similar kinds of loss, or whether some people have experienced multiple losses.

B. Identify common experiences.

Ask if people can see similarities between the different experiences of loss that have been listed. Are the feelings people express similar? Are their behaviors in response to loss similar? As the group expands on these ideas during the discussion, try to emphasize, when appropriate, that people often respond to different kinds of loss in similar ways.

Participants may describe a number of common grief reactions. They may report feeling sad, angry, hopeless or helpless, fearful, or numb. Often people who are grieving experience changes in appetite or sleep patterns. Sometimes people engage in self-destructive behaviors or actions that damage property or relationships. Strong feelings of grief may be expressed through a loss of interest in usual activities or a sense that life has no meaning or purpose.

C. Normalize grief reactions.

Loss and grieving are normal parts of life. People cannot arrange their lives so that they never experience loss.

5. The Current Situation of Loss

A. What's happening right now?

Review again the reason you are having this special session: someone the participants know is ill, and may be close to death; or someone they know has recently died.

B. Relate this to past experiences.

Ask people to look at the things that have been written on the butcher paper. Are the feelings they are having right now about this situation similar to or different from the other feelings that have been discussed today?

It is important to be completely accepting of what people say. Do not judge or compare people's statements. Often, it is helpful for people simply to talk about grief and sadness and to get no other response than the careful listening of others. Encourage and support this kind of sharing.

C. Talk about what's special in this situation.

This is a situation where someone close to participants has HIV disease. Is this different in any way from the other kinds of loss and grief people have experienced? Possible differences include:

- Participants might be afraid; for example, they might fear their own general risk of being HIV infected, and their specific risk of getting HIV from the person who is sick or who has died.* Participants may feel some special sadness about the death of someone "in the prime of his or her life."
- Participants may feel they have had to deal with other issues in addition to grief. For example, they may have dealt with feelings about homosexuality, drug use, and the stigma of AIDS.
- Participants may not feel free to talk about their true feelings. They may fear other people's reactions or prejudices regarding HIV disease.
- If the person who is ill has been a strong presence in the recovery program, participants may feel especially betrayed by his or her illness. "We need people like that as role models; it isn't fair to lose someone this important so early in recovery."

6. A Note about the Person Who Is Ill

A. Talk about what it is like to face illness.

If the ill person is still living, consider talking about how people interact with this person. Are they speaking honestly and openly with him or her? Are they avoiding the person? Are they being direct about recovery issues—their own and those of the ill person—or are they backing off from any confrontations? Are they letting the person deal with the situation in his or her own way, without pushing their own beliefs and attitudes?

People who have life-threatening illnesses cope in different ways. Some expect to die of their disease and can talk about this openly. Others are fighting the disease and expect to survive. Still others are uncomfortable talking about the illness or possible death.

---

* Even though HIV is not casually transmitted, many people are afraid of contracting the virus simply from being close to people who are infected. While it is important for participants to acknowledge and talk about these fears, it is also important for them to understand that these feelings are not based on fact.

People with HIV disease are often dealing with poor self image and loss of self-esteem. For example, someone who was once active and athletic may be unable to climb a set of stairs without becoming exhausted. Someone who was once witty and clever might have trouble speaking and remembering simple things. Some people with HIV disease feel guilty or angry about being infected; others are resigned to the situation. Many people with HIV disease have different feelings at different times about the illness.

People coping with serious illness must make their own decisions about how they see themselves in relation to the illness. Participants need to be honest about their feelings with their HIV-infected friends, but more importantly, they need to listen carefully when their friends want to talk and respect the silences when they do not.

7. Check in with the Group

A. Ask the group: "How are you doing with this discussion?"

B. Remind the group: "Talking about these feelings may stimulate responses you associate with drinking."

Participants may want to take a moment to think about their feelings. It is important for each to acknowledge if they feel an urge to drink in response to these powerful feelings and to seek ways of coping that will help them maintain sobriety.

8. Recovery: New Ways to Cope

A. Ask the group: "Other than drinking, what are some ways people can cope with their feelings about this situation?"

"Coping" does not mean getting rid of feelings. It means allowing the feelings to exist, acknowledging them, and staying sober and healthy even while the feelings are there. It is okay to have feelings that feel "bad."

Try to get several different answers from participants. You can give some of your own if the group does not come up with answers. Possible coping styles include:

- Talk to others about their feelings.

- Go to a meeting and listen to the experience, strength, and hope of others.
- Talk to your sponsor.
- Write in your journal.
- Exercise, even if it's just taking a walk around the block.
- Read literature that helps people understand more about how to cope with their feelings.

9. Closure

A. Sobriety is the most important thing in your life.

Grieving is hard. It is not a reason to go out and drink. Encourage participants to engage in healthy activities that will help them cope with difficult feelings, and remind them that this is some of the most important work in recovery.

Encourage people to talk to others about any feelings or thoughts they may have about today's session. Be available to talk to them yourself if possible.

HANDOUTS

The following section includes the handouts mentioned in the training sessions in this appendix. Among these are:

- "Using Condoms."
- "More about Using Condoms."
- "Using Latex Barriers."
- "Cleaning Needles and Works."
- "Safe and Unsafe Sexual Activities."

You may want to reproduce these handouts for use in these trainings. You may also want to enlarge them so that they fill an 8-1/2 inch by 11 inch page.

USING CONDOMS

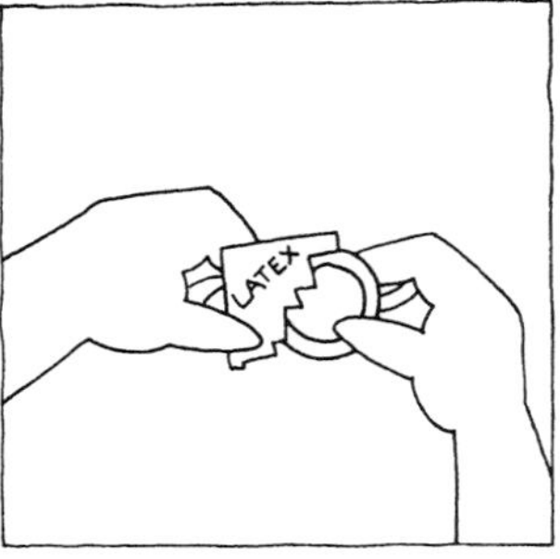

1. Use latex condoms. Open package carefully.

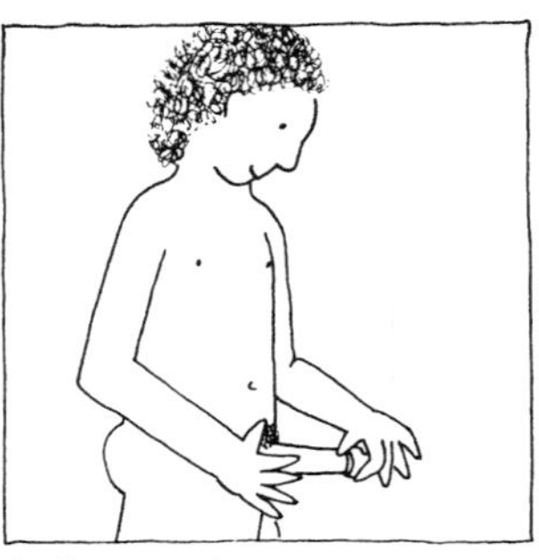

2. Put condom on erect (hard) penis.

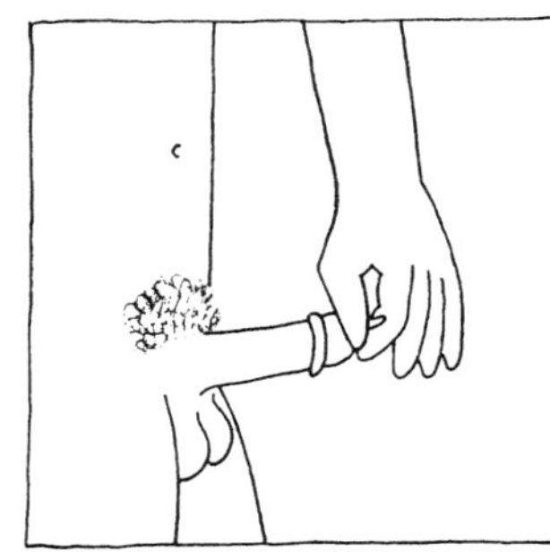

3. Press air out of tip of condom.

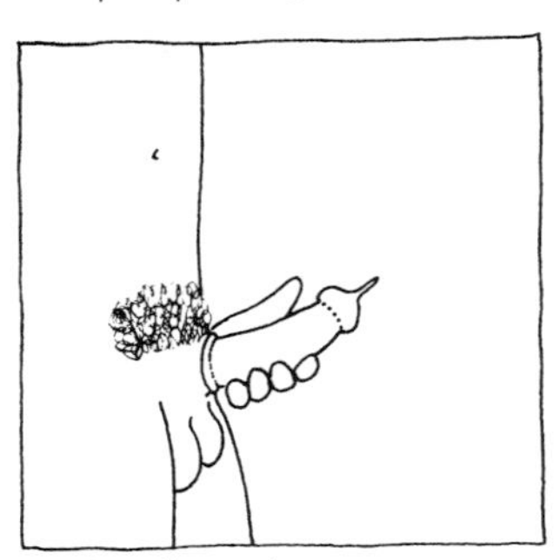

4. Unroll condom and cover whole penis.

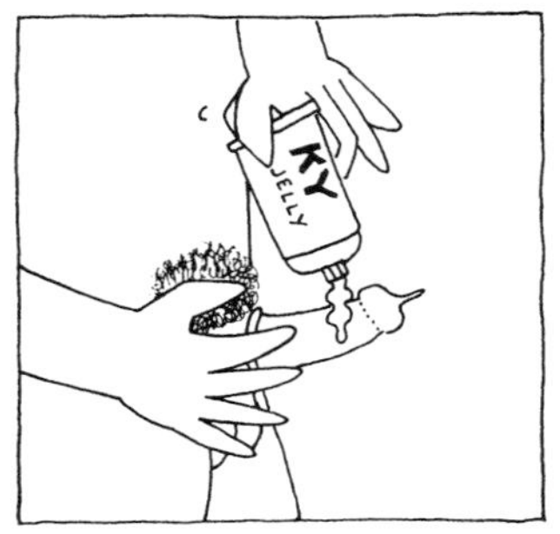

5. Always use water-based lubricant to help keep condom from breaking. Never use oil-based lubricants.

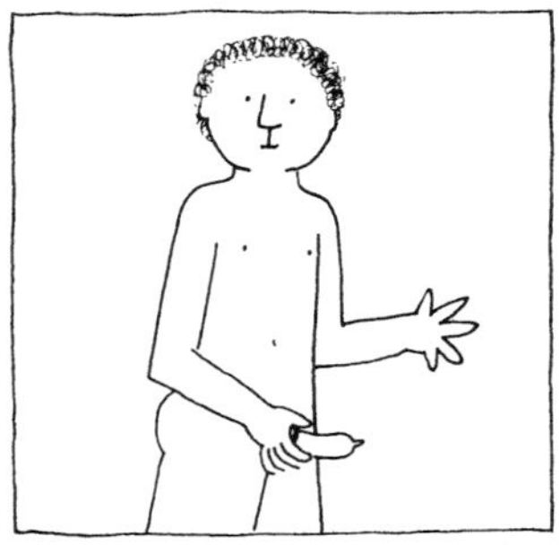

6. Hold condom at base during insertion.

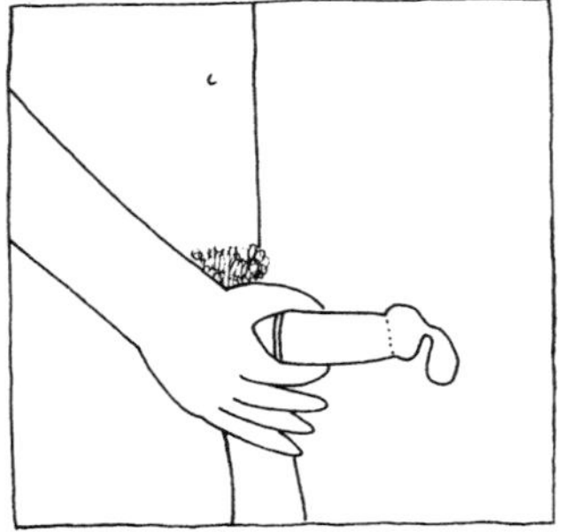

7. After sex, hold condom at base and pull out gently before penis gets soft.

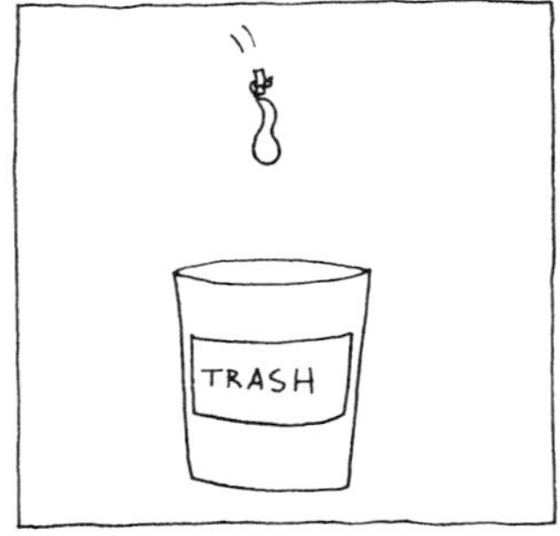

8. Use a condom only once and then throw away. Throw into trash, not down toilet.

From Quackenbush M, Benson JD, Rinaldi J. *Risk and Recovery: AIDS, HIV and Alcohol.* San Francisco: UCSF AIDS Health Project, 1992.

MORE ABOUT USING CONDOMS

Instructions for condom use are simple, but must be followed carefully. The main reason condoms fail is "user error." When people understand how to use condoms correctly, problems are rare.

1. Keep them handy. Keep a supply of condoms that are easy to get to "every time."
2. Store them properly. Keep condoms in a cool, dry place. The latex will break down more quickly in heat or sunlight. Condoms have a limited shelf life, so if you haven't used them after a few months, you should replace them.
3. Do not test condoms by inflating or stretching them. Condoms are electronically tested during manufacture. Stretching a condom increases the chances it will break.
4. Use a latex condom every time you have intercourse—vaginal, anal, or oral. Natural skin condoms do not protect as well against disease transmission.
5. Open the package carefully. Rough handling can damage condoms.
6. With thumb and forefinger, gently press any air out of the tip of the condom. Air bubbles can cause condoms to break. A dab of lubricant in the tip of the condom will solve the air problem and increase sensation for the person wearing the condom.
7. Unroll the condom so it covers the entire erect (hard) penis. If using a plain-ended condom (without a tip), leave about a half inch of condom free at the tip to catch the ejaculation. If uncircumcised, pull the foreskin back before putting on the condom. If the penis is erect, the condom will fit better. If the condom does not fit completely to the bottom of a man's penis, he should be careful not to insert beyond the condom base as this can cause the condom to come off.
8. Use plenty of water-soluble lubricant on the outside of the condom. Lubricant can also be put around vagina or anus before entry. Areas that are too dry can pull condoms off and tear them. Never use oil-based lubricants like *Crisco* or *Vaseline;* they can cause condom breakage in a few seconds! Do not use lubricants for oral sex: they taste terrible.
9. Hold onto the base of the condom when necessary, so the condom won't slip off. If the penis is getting soft, or a partner is very tight, the condom may slip. Certain sexual positions also tend to cause slipping. For example, when a partner is sitting on top of a man's penis, the vagina or anus may lift the condom.
10. After ejaculation, hold the condom around the base to avoid spilling contents or losing condom inside partner. Withdraw gently, while the penis is still partly erect.
11. Throw used condoms away! Condoms should not be used more than once. Never go from one person to another without changing condoms.
12. Practice, practice, practice! Condom use gets better with practice, and practice decreases the chances condoms will break and increases the likelihood of an enjoyable sexual experience. Users can practice with condoms while masturbating alone or engaging in other activities with a partner (mutual masturbation, fantasy).

USING LATEX BARRIERS

1. Latex dams are flat squares of latex rubber. They can be placed against a woman's vagina during mouth-to-vagina sex, or against a woman's or man's anus during mouth-to-anus sex. The dam keeps fluids from being shared between sex partners. It is believed latex dams can prevent HIV and other sexually transmitted diseases. To make a dam, cut down a non-lubricated condom so it lies flat. Or buy dental dams from dental supply houses or stores that sell sexual supplies.

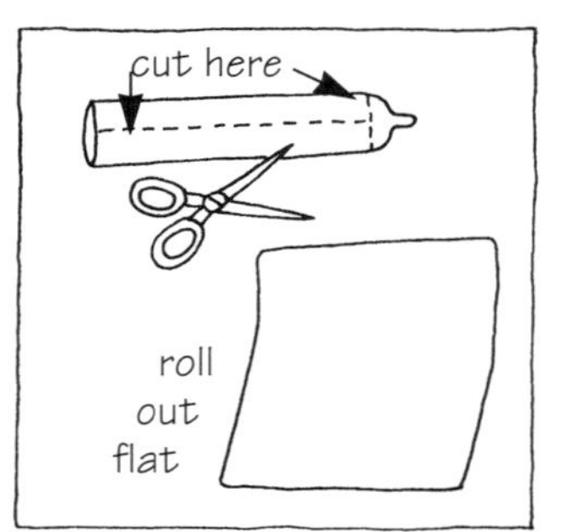

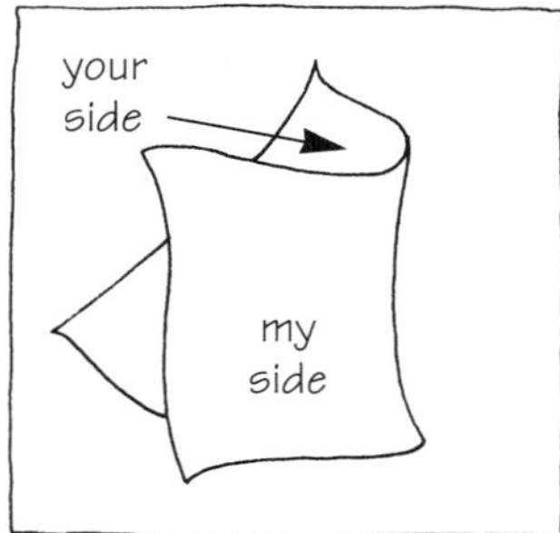

2. Be sure to keep one side towards you and the other side towards your partner.

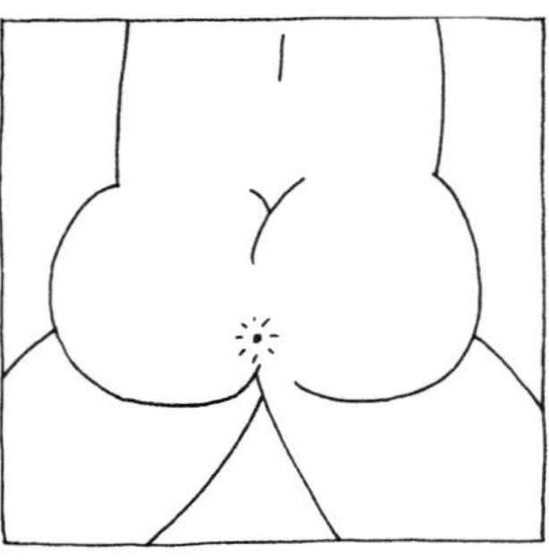

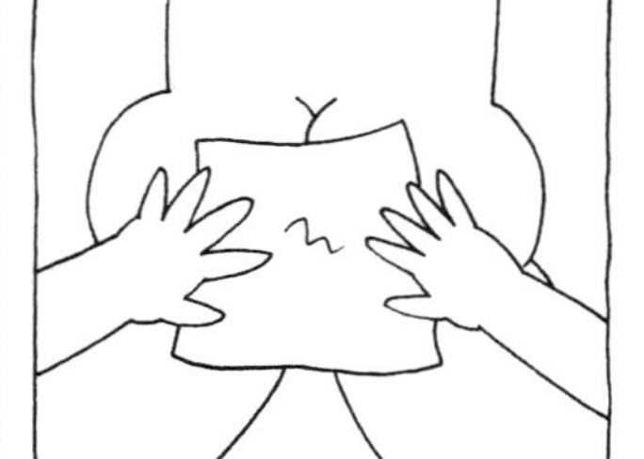

3. Place the dam over the anus for mouth-to-anus sex.

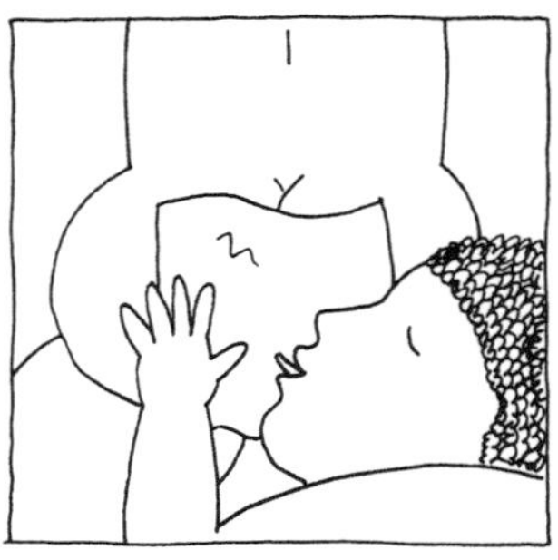

4. Don't use the same dam for anal, and then vaginal, sex.

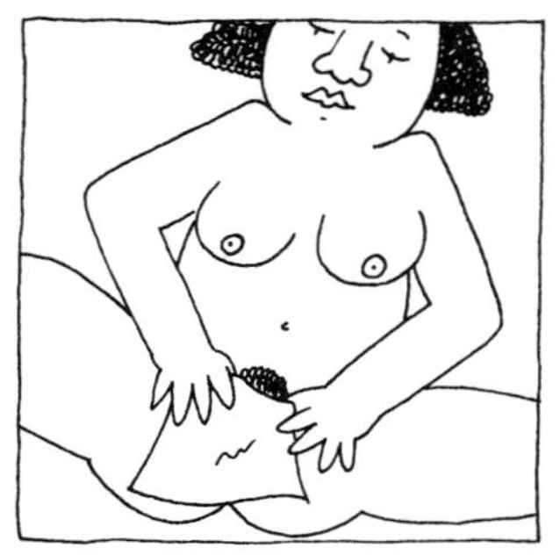

5. Place the dam over the vaginal lips for mouth-to-vagina sex.

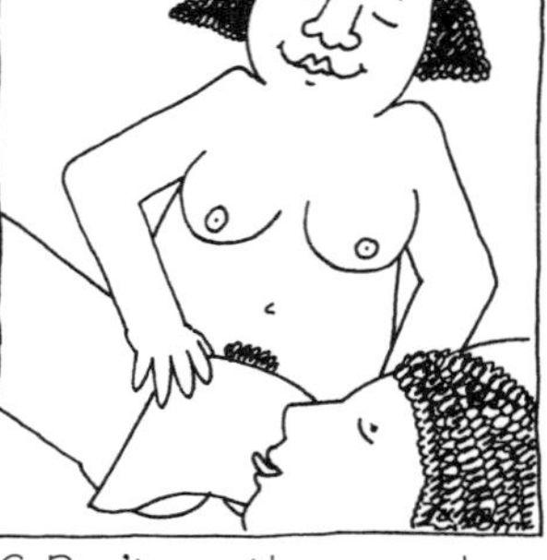

6. Don't use the same dam for anal, and then vaginal, sex.

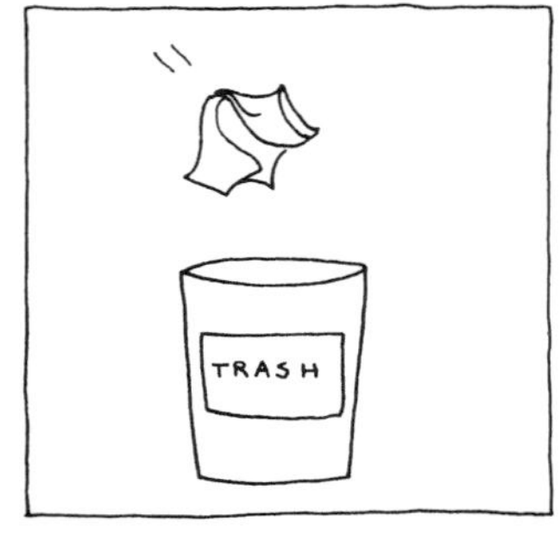

7. Use a latex dam only once and then throw away. Throw into trash, not down toilet.

From Quackenbush M, Benson JD, Rinaldi J. *Risk and Recovery: AIDS, HIV and Alcohol.* San Francisco: UCSF AIDS Health Project, 1992.

CLEANING NEEDLES AND WORKS

1. Best choice: Don't use needles at all.
2. Next best: Don't ever share needles or works with anybody for any reason.
3. Third choice: If you must share, always clean needles and works with bleach. Never share cottons. Never drink or shoot the bleach.

FIRST WITH BLEACH:

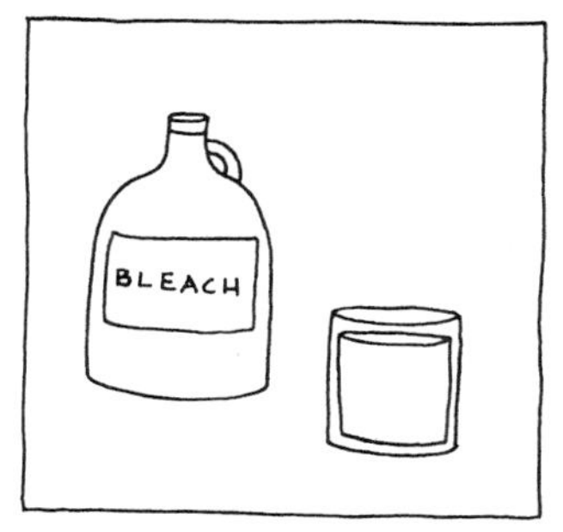

1. Pour liquid bleach (like Clorox) into a cup.

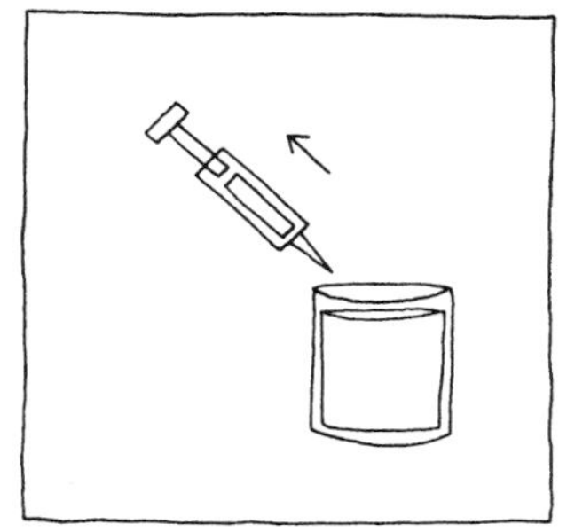

2. Fill syringe with bleach.

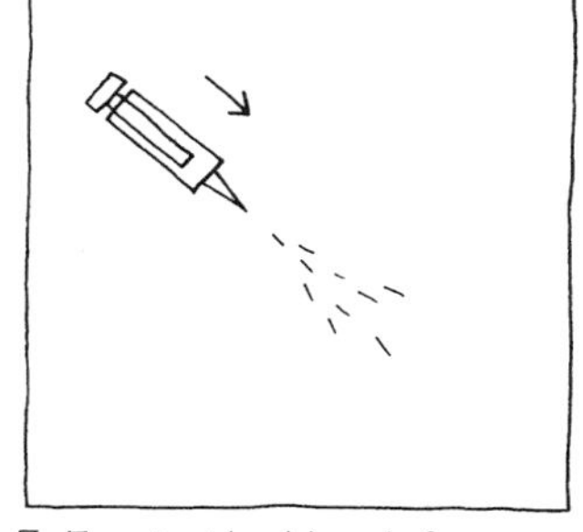

3. Empty the bleach from the syringe into sink or on the ground.
4. REPEAT these steps.

THEN WITH WATER:

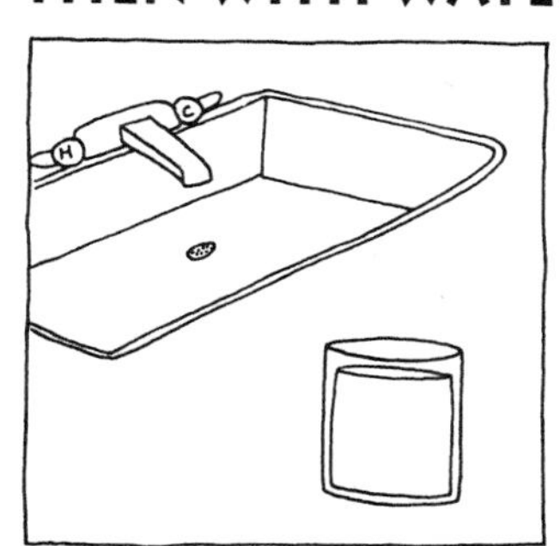

5. Fill cup with clean water.

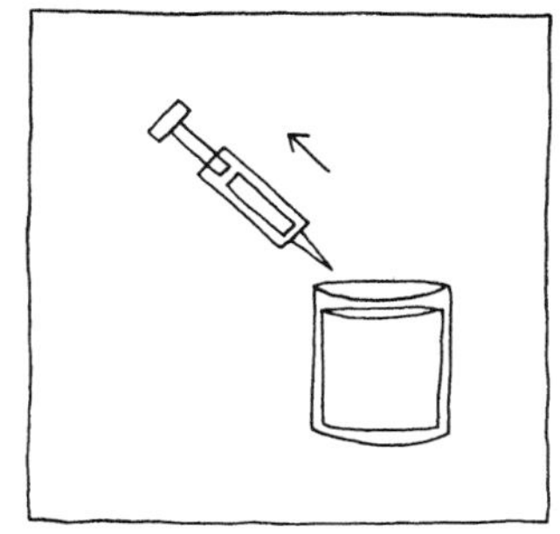

6. Fill syringe with water.

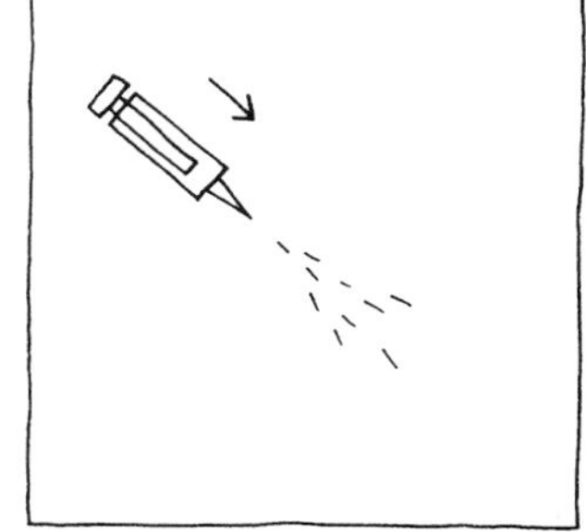

7. Empty the water from the syringe into sink or on ground.
8. REPEAT these steps.

From Quackenbush M, Benson JD, Rinaldi J. *Risk and Recovery: AIDS, HIV and Alcohol.* San Francisco: UCSF AIDS Health Project, 1992.

SAFE AND UNSAFE SEXUAL ACTIVITIES

Definitely Safe: No sharing of semen, vaginal secretions, or blood.

- Touching, massaging, hugging.
- Masturbation, alone or with someone else.
- Rubbing bodies together.
- Social (dry) kissing on the mouth.
- Kissing or licking the body: clean skin; no open sores; no mouth contact with genitals.
- Talking about sex, sharing fantasies.

Probably Safe: Probably no sharing of semen, vaginal secretions, or blood.

- Vaginal intercourse with a condom on the penis.*
- Oral intercourse on a man with a condom on the penis.*
- Oral intercourse on a woman with a latex barrier over the vulva
- Anal intercourse with a condom on the penis.*
- French kissing (wet) with no sores or cuts in either person's mouth.

In order to be safe, condoms must be properly used, and may not slip or break.

Definitely Unsafe: Sharing of semen, vaginal secretions, or blood.

- Vaginal intercourse without a condom.
- Anal intercourse without a condom.
- Any intercourse with a condom that slips, leaks, or breaks.
- Sharing objects put into the anus or vagina.
- Any activity that allows blood-to-blood contact, or allows blood contact with the mouth, vagina, or anus.

Other Considerations

- Oral sex is considered by some to be less risky than other activities such as anal or vaginal sex. Expert opinion ranges from "definitely unsafe" to "probably safe," however, there are HIV-infected people whose only HIV-related risk has been oral sex.
- Body fluids such as feces, nasal secretions, sputum, sweat, tears, urine, and vomit are not considered risky unless they contain visible blood.
- Breast milk, in a few cases, has transmitted HIV from mother to child. Precautions should be followed with breast milk.
- Saliva, which has been thoroughly studied, has never been shown to transmit HIV. It is not considered risky—but, see above, "French kissing."

From Quackenbush M, Benson JD, Rinaldi J. *Risk and Recovery: AIDS, HIV and Alcohol.* San Francisco: UCSF AIDS Health Project, 1992.

APPENDIX E

PROVIDER TRAINING TOOLS

HIV-related trainings support providers in learning new information and applying new skills to their interactions with participants. Workplace administrators cannot reasonably expect staff to approach HIV-related issues willingly and effectively if they are not properly trained in how to deal with these issues.

To help providers prepare to deal with HIV-related issues, a series of trainings might be scheduled over a period of several weeks or months. An initial training could cover basic information about HIV disease, including: how it is and is not transmitted, how to prevent transmission, the connection between HIV disease and alcohol, and the importance of providing HIV education in recovery programs. Additional trainings might cover the benefits of recovery for people with HIV disease, infection control guidelines, discussing the HIV antibody test with participants, supporting recovery participants with HIV disease, and exploring cultural issues likely to arise in HIV education and counseling.

Arranging and Developing Trainings

While it may take effort and creativity, arranging staff trainings will not necessarily cost additional money. Some communities already have resources for training in place. For example, local Department of Public Health staff may be able to address issues of infection control or describe local epidemiologic trends. Local AIDS agency staff or volunteers may be able to review basic HIV-related information. Within the local recovery community, people with HIV disease may be willing to talk to recovery staff about their experiences, and there may be providers knowledgeable about counseling issues who can describe some of the common concerns of people with HIV infection.

Materials in this book can help in the development of trainings for recovery staff. For example, the information in Chapter 1: *HIV and Alcohol: What's the Connection?* provides the background necessary to create a training introducing the topic of HIV disease to recovery providers. Chapter 4: *Facts about HIV Disease* provides a considerable resource of information that could be used to develop a training on HIV basics.

The information in Appendix C: *Infection Control* could be presented along with relevant case vignettes. This would establish an excellent foundation for a training on infection control guidelines. Such a training might include vignettes involving a participant who cuts his hand while preparing dinner; a participant who "borrows" someone else's razor, and then discovers that person has HIV disease; or an early morning support group during which one participant, after complaining of being ill, vomits, and group participants refuse to clean up because they are fearful they might contract HIV infection.

If you are developing your own training, keep in mind that people learn best by doing, that is, by participating in some activity that helps them learn the materials. In addition, they are more motivated to learn if they understand the rationale behind the training: why is it important for them to learn about this issue?

The four "Participant Education Sessions" included in these appendices can, with minor adaptation, also be useful for staff. These sessions cover HIV disease and safer sex, the use of condoms and latex barriers, deciding whether to take the HIV antibody test, and dealing with issues of grief and loss.

The following outline on "Exploring and Understanding Cultural Norms" was developed specifically for staff inservices. This outline is based on a training that has been provided successfully in dozens of settings.

SESSION #1 – EXPLORING AND UNDERSTANDING CULTURAL NORMS

OVERVIEW

TIME. 60 to 75 minutes.

PURPOSE. To help staff understand some of the barriers that may arise in HIV-related work with people from cultures different from their own.

TRAINEE KNOWLEDGE. Review of HIV basics would be helpful. See any of the participant education sessions in Appendix D: *Participant Training Tools* for an outline of this information.

MATERIALS. Collect the following materials for use during this session:

- Butcher paper.
- Markers.
- Masking tape.
- List of discussion questions for small group activities. (See page 230. Make one copy of each list for each small group.)

PREPARATION. Read the "Rationale" at the beginning of this outline. Read the full outline carefully before providing the training.

SUGGESTIONS FOR THIS SESSION. The learning in this module is based primarily on personal reflection and shared discussion. Facilitators should provide as much opportunity as possible for staff in the training to speak.

Some sections of the outline are presented in quotation marks. These are offered as suggested ways of explaining the material. You do not need to use these quotations in the training. In fact, your facilitation will be more effective if you use your own words and speak in a natural way.

Rationale

In discussing HIV disease with participants, providers often find themselves discussing topics that are challenging, difficult, or sensitive, topics like sexuality, homosexuality, drug use, illness, and death.

Everyone has his or her own ways of talking about such matters. Some of what a person knows about these issues or about how to discuss them is determined by his or her culture. When providers discuss such topics with people from cultures different from their own, there is a greater chance of misunderstanding or poor communication.

The activities in this training help staff look at their own cultural backgrounds and norms. This will help them understand more about issues likely to arise when working with participants who are culturally different from themselves.

The hour spent on this training is only a beginning exploration of the issues of cultural difference. It is not the goal of the training, nor is it within the capabilities of this activity, to address cultural concerns fully. It is hoped that the training will motivate staff to continue learning about themselves, and about cultural issues and differences.

Procedure

Introduction (5 minutes)

1. Framing. "In the course of our work, most of us deal with people who are different from ourselves in some way. For example, they may be of a different ethnic background, gender, sexual orientation, race, or age.

"When we talk with people about HIV disease, we must talk about matters that are difficult or sensitive—sexuality, illness, drug use, death, and homosexuality. In this activity, we'll look at some of the ways we use our own cultural backgrounds to define 'normal' ways to do things. We'll also think about how our own sense of cultural norms might complicate our work with people who have a different set of norms."

2. Limitations. Explain the limitations of this activity: "We do not expect to teach you all you need to know about counseling someone culturally different from you. We will not teach you attitudes, beliefs, behaviors, or facts about specific cultures. These are important things to learn about, however, and we hope our work here today will encourage you to learn more about these issues in the future."

3. Defining culture. In thinking about HIV-related work, it is useful to use a broad definition of culture. Culture is a group's "design for living"—the common assumptions about what is and what is not important, goals and meaning in life, what is right and what is wrong, how to behave and how to expect others to behave.

Discuss this definition briefly. Some important points to cover include:

- Culture is not the same thing as ethnicity or race. Culture is influenced by factors such as gender, class, educational experience, sexual orientation, political affiliations, and career.
- Cultures are not stagnant. They change in response to history, the environment, and the development of new ideas and values.
- Individuals within a culture may have values or behaviors that are different from others in the culture as a result of personal experiences. For example, someone who only likes meat and potatoes can develop a passion for Caesar salad. Or someone who believes drinking a lot of alcohol is a trait of culture—"I'm French, and all the French drink a lot"—can shift thinking and believe his or her own drinking is the result of a progressive disease.

Crossing cultural thresholds (10 minutes)

1. Cultural thresholds. The places where cultures differ can be thought of as "cultural thresholds." Everyone can cross certain thresholds easily, others with more difficulty. What is easy and what is difficult will vary from person to person.

2. Crossing cultural thresholds. Ask people to take a moment to think about whether the following cultural thresholds are easy or difficult for them to cross. How comfortable are they with

someone who is very different from them in each of the following areas? Then read the following list, slowly, giving people several seconds to consider each threshold:

- Sexual orientation
- Class
- Political
- Religious or spiritual
- Educational
- Ethnic
- Race
- Gender
- Age
- Beliefs about recovery

3. Discuss briefly. Did people find it easier or harder to think about crossing some of these thresholds? Invite people to share personal examples.

4. Crossing in different directions. Ask people whether they can cross a threshold more easily in one direction than another. For example, a middle class woman who identifies class as a difficult threshold might find it easier to cross that threshold with a person who is upper class than with someone who is poor or working class. Read over the list again, slowly.

5. Discuss briefly. Did people find differences? Invite people to share a personal example? Often, difficulty in one arena may reflect difficulties or ease in another. For example, for the same middle class woman who had difficulty crossing class thresholds, it might be more difficult to cross towards a working class man than towards a working class woman, which suggests some further issues about the threshold of gender.

Discovering some of our own norms (35 minutes)

1. Break up into small groups. Ask people to break into small groups with about four people in each group. In this activity, a group of three or a group of five will also work.

2. Explain the activity. Explain that one person in each group will need to volunteer to be the first "speaker" for this activity. The speakers will share some information about the culture in which they grew up and the culture they define as their own right now. Then other people in the small group will talk about similarities and differences in their own cultures, past and present.

3. Select speakers. Ask each group to identify a speaker for the first topic.

4. First topic: Sex. The speakers should start by taking a minute or two to define their culture: first, the culture they identified with when they were growing up, and then the culture they identify with now.

Then the speakers can talk about sex. "In the culture in which you grew up, how did you talk about sex? What words did you use? Who could you talk to about sex? How were you expected to learn about sexual matters? What feelings were you supposed to have about sex? What beliefs? What was the purpose of sex? You can mention anything else that comes up as you share this information." Hand out the list of these discussion questions to the speaker in each group. (See page 230.)

Other people in the group should listen to what the speaker has to say without interrupting or asking questions. Ask them, as they listen, to think about their own cultures—both as they currently define them and as they did while growing up—and whether their belief systems are similar to or different from the speaker's. Let the groups know that the speakers will talk for seven to eight minutes and that further instructions will follow.

5. Small group discussion. After seven to eight minutes, stop the speakers, and invite the small groups to discuss among themselves the differences between the cultural norms of their speaker and those of the listeners. This is the time for listeners to talk about what it was like for them when they grew up and how it is now. Tell the groups they will have seven to eight minutes for their discussions.

6. Second speaker. After about seven to eight minutes, ask the

groups to close and to identify a second speaker. Make sure all the groups have a speaker identified.

7. SECOND TOPIC: DEATH. As above, the second speaker should start with a brief definition of his or her own culture, past and present.

Then the speaker should talk about death. "How was death viewed in the culture in which you grew up? Did your family or friends know anyone who had died? How were people supposed to react to someone's death? If you had questions, who could you talk to? What were children supposed to know and understand about death? You can mention anything else that comes up as you share this information. Hand out the list of these discussion questions to speakers in each group. (See page 230.) Remind the groups that the speakers will have seven to eight minutes to talk.

8. SMALL GROUP DISCUSSION. Once again, after seven to eight minutes, stop the speakers, and invite the small groups to discuss among themselves the differences between the cultural norms of the speaker and those of the listeners. This discussion should last seven to eight minutes.

DISCUSSION AND CONCLUSIONS (10-15 MINUTES)

1. PREPARE FOR GROUP DISCUSSION. Prepare the full group for a discussion of the training activities, but ask people to remain seated with their small groups.

2. DEFINING DIFFERENCES IN WORKING WITH CLIENTS. "We've defined culture broadly in this activity. Using that broad definition, what kinds of differences do you find between yourselves and the program participants you work with? For example, are clients of different religions, ages, or races?"

3. NORMS ABOUT HIV DISEASE AND AIDS. "In your work, as you talk with people of different backgrounds about HIV disease and AIDS, what differences in norms or expectations are likely to surface? Or, if you have done this kind of education already, what differences have surfaced?"

4. Responses. Ask the small groups to discuss how to respond to these differences in ways that will help strengthen HIV-related education and counseling. They might think about ways to build trust, increase a participant's understanding of HIV-related facts, or encourage someone to make changes in behavior to protect his or her health. Each group should come up with one suggested response to share with the full group. (If there are only two small groups, you may want to invite each group to come up with two suggested responses.)

5. Sharing ideas. After five minutes, ask groups to share their ideas and suggestions. You might want to write some of these suggestions down on butcher paper.

6. Conclusion. Differences in values, language, and beliefs are inevitable. It is essential to keep these differences in mind, and to do the best job to bridge the gaps created by these differences.

CULTURAL NORMS

QUESTIONS ABOUT SEX

Think about and discuss the following questions.

- In the culture in which you grew up, how was sex talked about?
- What words did people use to refer to sexual activities or sexual parts?
- When you were young, who could you talk to about sex?
- How were you expected to learn about sexual matters?
- What feelings were you supposed to have about sex? What beliefs?
- What was the purpose of sex?

Mention anything else that comes up as you share this information.

QUESTIONS ABOUT DEATH

Think about and discuss the following questions.

- How was death viewed in the culture in which you grew up?
- Did you, your family, or friends know anyone who had died?
- How were people supposed to react to someone's death?
- Who could you talk to if you had questions about death?
- What were children supposed to know and understand about death?

Mention anything else that comes up as you share this information.

APPENDIX F

AIDS AND ALCOHOL ORGANIZATIONS

AIDS Organizations

National AIDS Hotline, Centers for Disease Control (CDC)
(800) 342-AIDS; (800) 344-SIDA (Spanish language);
(800) AIDS-TTY (TDD/TTY for hearing impaired)
Answers to questions about AIDS and HIV disease; information about and referrals to AIDS organizations, local resource centers, and local AIDS hotlines; pamphlets and other written materials.

National AIDS Information Clearinghouse (NAIC)
P.O. Box 6003, Rockville, MD 20849-6003
(800) 458-5231
Information about AIDS organizations; information about federal and state education and treatment programs; pamphlets and other written materials.

Project Inform
1965 Market Street, Suite 220, San Francisco, CA 94103
(800) 822-7422; (800) 334-7422 (California)
Information about approved, experimental, and alternative treatments for HIV disease; newsletter.

Alcohol Organizations

Al-Anon Family Groups
P.O. Box 682, Midtown Station, New York NY 10018
(212) 302-7240
Support and help for family and friends of alcoholics. Check telephone listings for local groups.

Alcoholics Anonymous World Services, Inc.
P.O. Box 459, Grand Central Station, New York, NY 10163
(212) 870-3400
Support and help for alcoholics. Check telephone listings for local groups.

National Council on Alcoholism and Drug Dependence
(800) 475-HOPE
Information and education concerning alcoholism and drug dependence.

FURTHER READING

Alcoholics Anonymous. *Alcoholics Anonymous.* New York: Alcoholics Anonymous World Services, Inc., 1992.

Alcoholics Anonymous. *Twelve Steps and Twelve Traditions.* New York: Alcoholics Anonymous World Services, Inc., 1991.

Baker RA, Moulton JM, Tighe J. *Early Care for HIV Disease.* (2nd edition). San Francisco: San Francisco AIDS Foundation, 1992.

Mann J. *AIDS in the World in 1992.* Cambridge: Harvard University Press. Forthcoming.

Metzger L. *From Denial to Recovery: Counseling Problem Drinkers, Alcoholics, and Their Families.* San Francisco: Jossey-Bass Publishers, 1988.

Mikluscak-Cooper, Miller EE. *Living in Hope: A 12-Step Approach for Persons at Risk or Infected with HIV.* Berkeley, Calif.: Celestial Arts, 1991.

Tilleraas P. *Circle of Hope: Our Stories of AIDS, Addiction and Recovery.* Center City, Minn.: Hazelden, 1990.

Tilleraas P. *The Color of Light: Daily Meditations for All of Us Living with AIDS.* Center City, Minn.: Hazelden, 1988.

GLOSSARY

12-step program. Self-help programs based on the Twelve Steps of Alcoholics Anonymous. AA is the best-known and most widely used of all 12-step programs. Other programs include Al-Anon (for families and friends of alcoholics), Narcotics Anonymous (for drug addicts), Overeaters Anonymous, and Debtors Anonymous.

Addiction. Physical or psychological dependence on alcohol or other drugs. Often includes an overwhelming involvement with acquiring and using a substance, an inability to stop using, and a tendency to start using after periods of abstinence.

AIDS. Acquired immunodeficiency syndrome, a viral disease that results in impairment of the body's immune system. People with AIDS can get a number of life-threatening diseases that do not affect individuals with healthy immune systems. They can also contract severe cases of more common diseases. AIDS is generally diagnosed at the most advanced stage of HIV infection, and this diagnosis signals significant damage to the body's immune system.

Antibody. Specialized protein manufactured by the body's immune system to help fight disease. Antibodies for different diseases vary in their effectiveness to fight those diseases. Antibodies to HIV appear to fight the infection for a period of time, but eventually falter and fail to protect the body.

Antibody test. A blood test that can detect the presence of HIV antibodies in the blood. A positive HIV antibody test indicates HIV infection. A negative antibody test indicates that no antibodies to HIV were found, and that the person is either uninfected or has been infected recently and has not yet developed antibodies (See also "window period").

Antibody testing is performed in anonymous or confidential settings. During anonymous testing, test-takers offer no identifying information, such as name, address, or phone number. Instead, they are usually given a code number at the time their blood is drawn, and offer that code number to receive their results. During confidential testing, test-takers provide identifying information thereby creating a record of the test. Confidentiality of these records is protected by the laws that protect medical records, and in some states or regions, by additional laws specific to HIV-related information.

ARC. "AIDS-related complex," a diagnosis that was once given to people infected with HIV, who showed symptoms of infection but did not meet criteria for an AIDS diagnosis. Generally this term is no longer used. The preferred term is "symptomatic HIV infection."

Body fluids; body substances. Any fluids or substances produced by the body. In the context of HIV disease, body substances considered to present some risk are blood, tissue, semen, vaginal secretions, breast milk, and any other fluid that has visible blood in it. Tears, sweat, saliva, sputum, nasal secretions, urine, feces, and vomit are not considered risky substances unless visible blood is present.

Blood transfusion. To take blood from one person (the donor) and transfer it to the vein of a second person (the recipient). In the past, HIV infection was transmitted through blood transfusions by donors who were unaware that they were infected. In the U.S., donated blood has been screened since 1985 using the HIV antibody test, and HIV transmission through blood transfusions is now very rare. There is no HIV-associated risk in donating blood.

Casual contact. Daily contact between people at home, school, work, or in the community, that does not involve sexual interactions or needle sharing. HIV is not transmitted through casual contact.

Centers for Disease Control (CDC). A federal agency that monitors the incidence of different diseases, ways diseases are transmitted, and treatments for disease. The CDC provides health and safety recommendations for health care workers and the general public.

Disinhibition. Loss of inhibitions. People who drink alcohol often experience disinhibiting effects, and find themselves engaging in behaviors that, when sober, they would not practice.

Early intervention. In the context of HIV disease, medical intervention—including antibody testing—early in the course of disease, often before symptoms develop. It may also involve provision of social or psychological support.

Epidemiology. The study of disease trends, especially how many people have a given disease, how they contracted the disease, what treatments they are using, and how effective the treatments are.

Hemophilia. A genetic disease in which the body is unable to manufacture factor VIII, a blood product produced by the body that aids in clotting after a bleeding injury. People with hemophilia can sometimes face serious, even life-threatening, circumstances as the result of minor cuts or bruises. Hemophilia has been treated with factor VIII manufactured from blood donations, and early on in the AIDS epidemic, many people with hemophilia became infected with HIV. Factor VIII is now manufactured in a way that prevents HIV transmission.

HIV. Human immunodeficiency virus, the virus that causes AIDS.

HIV infection; HIV disease. Anyone who has been infected with HIV is said to have HIV infection or HIV disease. These terms define a wide spectrum of medical circumstances ranging from healthy without symptoms of infection (often early in the course of disease) to severe and life-threatening symptoms (late in the course of infection). The course of disease often ranges to more than 12 years.

Homophobia. Unreasonable fear, dislike, or judgment of gay men or lesbians.

Immune system. The system that protects the body from foreign organisms and toxins.

Incubation period. The period of time from infection to the development of symptoms or the diagnosis of disease. In the context of HIV disease, it takes an average of six to eight years for a person to develop symptoms and an average of 10 years to develop an AIDS-defining disease (a disease that indicates an AIDS diagnosis).

Injection drug user (IDU). A person who injects drugs for recreational use into the veins or muscles, or under the skin.

Intravenous drug user (IVDU). A person who injects drugs for recreational use directly into the veins. Sometimes used interchangeably with "injection drug user," though technically the term does not include persons who inject drugs into the muscles or under the skin.

Inventory. In 12-step programs, an assessment of one's own behavior in a particular situation or throughout life. The inventory helps individuals define strengths and weaknesses in interpersonal interactions, and recognize their own role in their misfortunes and difficulties.

Kaposi's sarcoma (KS). A tumor of the blood or lymphatic vessel walls, sometimes seen in HIV-infected people. KS usually appears as pink or purple blotches on the skin.

Opportunistic infections. Infections that arise in individuals whose immune systems are compromised or damaged. These infections take advantage of the weakened immune system, hence the name "opportunistic."

Paraphernalia. In the context of injection drug use, any of the equipment used to prepare or inject drugs, including spoons (for heating and mixing drugs into a liquid form), cottons (for straining the mixture), syringes, and needles.

Person with AIDS (PWA); person with HIV disease (PWHIV). Preferred over terms such as "AIDS victim" or "AIDS patient." Supports people with HIV disease in perceiving themselves as active participants in treatment and healing, and acknowledges that they more than merely patients or cases of disease.

Pneumonia. Inflammation and infection of the lungs.

Pneumocystis carinii pneumonia (PCP). A type of pneumonia that only appears in individuals with impaired immune systems. One of the most common HIV-related opportunistic infections.

Post-test counseling. Counseling provided in the process of giving out HIV antibody test results. Usually emphasizes what results mean, plans for protecting future health, and strategies to avoid further HIV transmission.

Pre-test counseling. Counseling provided before someone has blood drawn for the HIV antibody test. Usually involves a description of the test and what information it provides, background on HIV-related risk activities, and an assessment of the test-taker's own risk situation and ways to decrease risk.

Reinfection. Subsequent occurrences of HIV transmission in people who are already HIV infected. This is dangerous, since HIV mutates quickly and exists in many different strains, and additional infections with different forms of the virus can speed up the progression of the disease.

Risk. Chance of injury, damage, or loss.

Safe needle use. Use of needles for injection drugs in a manner that will not transmit HIV. The preferred approach is not to share needles or injection equipment for any purpose. Another choice is to clean needles and equipment with bleach before sharing.

Safer sex. Sexual activities that carry little or no risk of transmitting HIV. These include behaviors in which risky body fluids—blood, semen, and vaginal secretions—are not exchanged between sexual partners.

Semen. The thick, whitish fluid secreted by males at the point of sexual orgasm: "Cum."

Seroconvert. To shift, or "convert," from being uninfected to being HIV infected. To develop detectable levels of HIV antibody after HIV infection.

Seropositive. In the case of HIV disease, the condition of having HIV antibodies detected in the blood. Having HIV infection. "Seronegative" is the condition of having no HIV antibodies detected in the blood.

Serum. A clear, yellowish fluid that separates from a blood clot after coagulation. "Plasma" is the liquid portion of the blood, and serum is what is left of plasma after the process of coagulation removes a specific clotting agent.

Sexually transmitted disease (STD). Any of a number of diseases that are commonly spread through sexual activity. HIV infection is a sexually transmitted disease.

Slip. A relapse. In alcoholism, the alcoholic in recovery "slips" and takes a drink. In HIV disease, a person who has made a commitment to practice safer sex or needle use "slips" and engages in a risky activity.

Survivor guilt. A psychological state in which the survivor of a catastrophe feels guilty for surviving when others have died or been seriously injured. A common experience for people who test negative for HIV antibody but who have engaged in the same kinds of risks as their HIV-infected friends.

Tissue. A collection of similar, specialized cells that together perform a particular function, for example, skin tissue, muscle tissue, nerve tissue.

Transmission. The passage of a disease-causing organism—bacteria, virus, fungus—from one person to another.

Universal precautions. Standard infection control guidelines that should be practiced "universally" in first aid and medical treatment settings, that is, with all patients under all circumstances. These guidelines minimize the exposure of providers or patients to blood or body fluids, and limit the risk of HIV or other disease transmission.

Vaginal secretions. The natural lubrication or secretions of the vagina, including those produced during periods of sexual excitement.

Virus. An organism made up of genes surrounded by a protein coating. Technically, a virus is not actually a living organism because it cannot reproduce itself. It must invade a living cell to reproduce. Viruses are smaller than any living organism.

Vulva. The external genital organs of females. Includes the labia (lips), the clitoris, and the opening of the vagina.

Window period. The time period from the point of first infection with HIV to the development of measurable HIV antibodies. The window period usually runs two to 12 weeks and may last as long as six months and, in very rare cases, even longer. During the window period, an HIV-infected person may test HIV antibody negative.

Works. Equipment or paraphernalia used in injection drug use. Often called a "rig."

INDEX

RELATED PUBLICATIONS

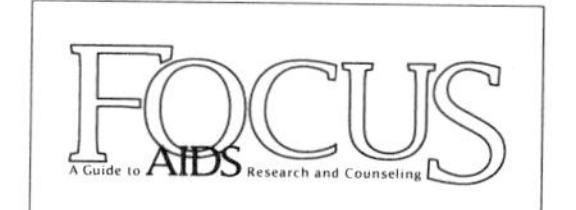

FOCUS: A Guide to AIDS Research and Counseling. This monthly newsletter reviews the counseling aspects of AIDS: how HIV-related counseling is affected by the medical, epidemiological, and social realities of AIDS, as well as the emotional response to the disease. Since 1985, FOCUS has been an indispensable reference for the 25,000 counselors, health providers, and scholars who read it.

Recent subjects have included: AIDS Counseling for Drug Injectors, the Dying Client, the Rural Epidemic, HIV-related Financial Issues, the Workplace Response to HIV Disease, Challenges Facing Women, and Early Intervention.

Face to Face
A Guide to AIDS Counseling

FACE TO FACE: A Guide to AIDS Counseling. This book presents an overview of the mental health and psychosocial aspects of AIDS. Fifty internationally recognized experts offer thoughtful and reliable information to help health professionals, care providers, and lay people counsel those at risk for or infected with HIV.

AIDS Law for Mental Health Professionals

AIDS Law for Mental Health Professionals (Updated Version). This book explores the legal and ethical issues confronting therapists when they treat people with concerns about HIV disease. Focusing on California law, the book discusses issues relevant to practitioners everywhere: the duty to treat, confidentiality, the duty to warn, suicide, and the responsibilities the of HIV-infected therapist. Although California law is not necessarily applicable in other states, it often serves as a model for AIDS law elsewhere. Includes subscription to *Judicious Practice,* a free, annual update newsletter.

AIDS'
Effects on the Brain

AIDS' Effects on the Brain. Prepared for families, friends, and caregivers, this brochure examines the neurological symptoms of HIV infection and offers helpful information on the management of patients with these problems.

ORDER FORM

Name ______________________ Daytime Phone (____) ____________

Title ______________________

Organization ______________________

Address ______________________

____

Counselor Trainings

AHP offers a variety of HIV-related trainings for providers.
Please check here if you are interested in more information about our trainings _____

To order additional titles:

Title		Price	x Quantity	= Total
AIDS Law for Mental Health Professionals	(book)	$ 19.95	____	______
Face to Face: A Guide to AIDS Counseling	(book)	$ 14.95	____	______
FOCUS individual subscription	(foreign = $ 48.00)	$ 36.00	____	______
FOCUS institutional subscription	(foreign = $ 110.00)	$ 90.00	____	______
AIDS' Effects on the Brain	(40¢ each for 26 or more)	$ .65	____	______
	Subtotal			______
Shipping, $3 first item, $1 add. items	*(not for FOCUS)*		____	______
Sales tax, California residents only		8.5 %	____	______
	Total			______

Payment

____ Check enclosed - payable to *AIDS Health Project*

____ Visa ____ Master Card Account number ______________________

Expiration date ____________ Signature ______________________

____ Bill me (net 30 days) Purchase order number ______________________

Signature ______________________

Mail to UCSF AIDS Health Project, Box 0884, San Francisco, CA, 94143-0884
For further information, please call (415) 476-6430